SPEECH AND LANGUAGE DISORDERS

HANDWRITING AND DYSGRAFIA

RELATION AND ASSESSMENT

SPEECH AND LANGUAGE DISORDERS

Additional books and e-books in this series can be found on Nova's website under the Series tab.

SPEECH AND LANGUAGE DISORDERS

HANDWRITING AND DYSGRAFIA

RELATION AND ASSESSMENT

MONIQUE HERRERA CARDOSO
AND
SIMONE APARECIDA CAPELLINI
EDITORS

nova
science publishers
New York

Library of Congress Cataloging-in-Publication Data

Names: Herrera Cardoso, Monique. | Aparecida Capellini, Simone.
Title: Handwriting and dysgrafia: relation and assessment / editors, Monique Herrera Cardoso and Simone Aparecida Capellini (Speech and Hearing Sciences Department, São Paulo State University "Júlio de Mesquita Filho", UNESP, Marbilia, São Paulo, Brazil).
Description: Hauppauge, New York: Nova Science Publisher's, Inc., [2018] | Series: Speech and language disorders | Includes bibliographical references and index.
Identifiers: LCCN 2018025724 (print) | LCCN 2018026053 (ebook) | ISBN 9781536138061 (ebook) | ISBN 9781536138054 (softcover) | ISBN 9781536138061 (ebook)
Subjects: LCSH: Agraphia. | Language disorders in children.
Classification: LCC RC429 (ebook) | LCC RC429 .H356 2018 (print) | DDC 616.85/53--dc23
LC record available at https://lccn.loc.gov/2018025724

Published by Nova Science Publishers, Inc. † New York

Contents

PREFACE

The book entitled *Handwriting and Dysgrafia: Relation and Assessment* is composed by nine chapters with scientific contributions in the fields of Speech Language Pathology, Education, Occupational Therapy, and Physical Education.

Capellini and Cardoso present the first chapter on *The Process of Acquisition and Development of Handwriting*. The second chapter is from Alves, Van Petten, Cardoso and Magalhães on *Transcultural Adaptation of the Here's How I Write (HHIW) for Brazilian Children.* Milani, Hiraga and Pellegrini wrote the third chapter on *Assessment of the Handwriting Quality: an Instrument for the Brazilian Educational Context.*

The fourth chapter is from Martins and Bastos on *Understanding, Diagnosis and Intervention in Dysgraphia.* Cardoso and Capellini present the fifth contribution on *Application of the Detailed Assessment of Speed of Handwriting (DASH) to Brazilian Students.* The sixth contribution is written by Cardoso, Liporaci and Capellini entitled *The Quality of Handwriting of Elementary School Students II: Comparison Between Boys and Girls.*

Damasceno, Arnaut, Marques and Avila present the seventh contribution on *Handwriting and Orthographic Learning. The Speed and Legibility of Handwriting of Dyslexic Students* is the eighth contribution by Cardoso, Santos and Capellini. The ninth chapter and final contribution entitled *Relationship Between Viso-motor Skills and Handwriting in Students with Dyslexia* is from the authors Capellini, Serrão, Del Bianco, Germano and Giaconi

I conclude this preface wishing a good reading on handwriting and dysgrafia for everyone!

Dr. Simone Aparecida Capellini
Department of Speech and Hearing Sciences
São Paulo State University "Júlio de Mesquita Filho" (UNESP)
Marília, São Paulo, Brazil

In: Handwriting and Dysgrafia
Editors: M. Herrera Cardoso et al.
ISBN: 978-1-53613-805-4

Chapter 1

THE PROCESS OF ACQUISITION AND DEVELOPMENT OF HANDWRITING

***Simone Aparecida Capellini, PhD*[1,*]**
***and Monique Herrera Cardoso*[2,†]**
[1]Department of Speech and Hearing Sciences,
São Paulo State University "Júlio de Mesquita Filho" (UNESP),
Marília, São Paulo, Brazil
[2] Education Program,
São Paulo State University "Júlio de Mesquita Filho" (UNESP),
Marília, São Paulo, Brazil

ABSTRACT

This chapter initially addresses the definition and function of writing, its relation to oral language and other skills necessary for its development, focusing on the requirements of the Brazilian Ministry of Education and the practices used by educational institutions. It also discusses the concept of dysgraphia and the characteristics of this

---

* Full-Professor; Corresponding Author: sacap@uol.com.br
† Graduate Student

diagnosis, given the importance of readability and speed of writing, besides characterizing the possible pathologies that may present this spectrum of dysgraphia. In addition, it presents a survey of studies and international instruments, which investigate the quality, and speed of handwriting, reinforcing the shortage of articles in Brazil, and it is concluded with important aspects to be taken into account during handwriting evaluation. It is expected that this chapter may help health and education professionals to elucidate how the process of acquiring and developing handwriting occurs, emphasizing its importance nowadays.

Keywords: manual writing, dysgraphia, education

THE HANDWRITING

Writing is a cultural invention, in which its earliest forms date back six thousand years. Its function is communication, playing the role of spreading culture and concepts of humanity (Planton, Jucla, Roux, & Demonet, 2013), thus, the act of writing consists on the ability of the subject to express thoughts and ideas, fundamental to success in school, in the labor market and for participation in modern society (Kim, Al Otaiba, & Wanzek, 2015).

However, in order to be able of writing properly, it is imperative to have developed oral language and phonology correctly. According to Miranda (2012, p. 129) "[...] writing is the means which allows the transposition of the sound system to the secondary substance, that is manifested into visible traces materialized on paper, or on a computer screen."

It is known that before completing seven years of age, Brazilian children must have acquired all the sounds of speech (Wertzner, 1995), a period in which the process of literacy begins, and school children are requested to recognize the letters visually, and perform letter coding/transcription according to their phonological correspondent (Whitehurst & Lonigan, 1998).

In order to be accurate on recording letter forms, the student will require fine motor skills, visual perception, perceptual-visual-motor integration, maturity and integration of cognition (Stevenson & Just, 2014), which makes the development of writing a long, demanding and complex process (Chang & Yu, 2013), requiring the involvement of different skills and many brain systems interacting dynamically, to produce the desired result (Vinci-Booher, James & James, 2016). In other words, the use of manual writing requires the visual mnemonic representations of each letter, the recognition of the traits which make up each letter and the ability to reproduce these traits in a sequential order and direction (Schickedanz, 1999).

A study realized with elementary school children (Overvelde & Hulstijn, 2011) found that handwriting develops rapidly during the first school year (ages 6 to 7), evolves around 7 to 8 years, and becomes automatic and organized around 8 to 9 years. From the moment the calligraphy becomes automatic, the writer no longer needs to focus consciously on the mechanics of writing, and consequently frees up work memory resources and attention to the high-level writing process (for example, the revision of the written text), thus guaranteeing a better written text (McCarney, Peters, Jackson, Thomas, & Kirby, 2013).

It is noteworthy that during the manual writing process, students acquire their own calligraphy style (Simonnet, Anquetil, & Bouillon, 2017), since their individual characteristics (such as gender, preferences, skill level and practice with writing, motor coordination, motivation, and others) may interfere on the quality and speed of writing (Ahmed, Rasool, Afzal, & Siddiqi, 2017).

However, on the initial series of literacy, teachers provide a model of graphic symbols. When the quality of the symbol written by the student does not correspond to the expectation of the teacher, i.e., the readability of the written material is impaired, and a more detailed investigation becomes necessary. In Brazil, the Program of Support to Reading and Writing - PRALER (Brazil, 2007), developed by the Ministry of Education, provides the models of letters that students should learn by the end of the 3rd grade of elementary school (Figure 1). However, the time spent practicing handwriting in subsequent school years depends on the criteria of each teaching institution.

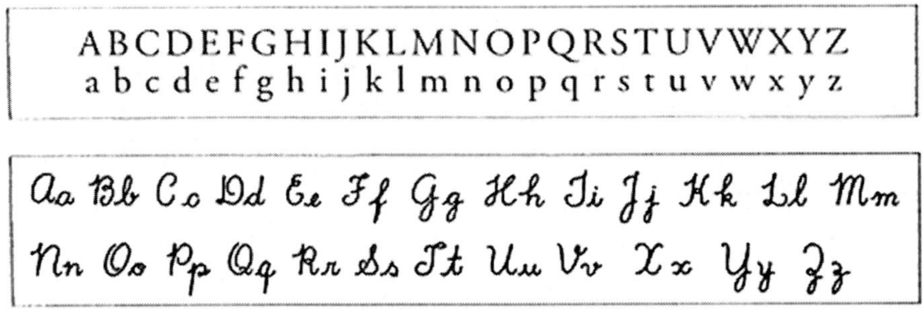

Source: PRALER, 2007.

Figure 1. Model of cursive letters and stick, lowercase and upper case suggested by the Brazilian Ministry of Education.

Therefore, the practice of handwriting is indispensable, since it allows the schoolchildren to reduce their working memory requirements as quickly as possible (Sampaio & Cardoso, 2015). However, even with adequate practice, the literature points out that about 5% to 30% of school-aged-children may present difficulties with the development of handwriting (Duiser, Van Der Kamp, Ledebt, & Savelsbergh, 2014, Overvelde & Hulstijn, and consequently tend to be frustrated when trying to put their ideas on the paper, inhibiting their ability to compose texts (Medwell & Wray, 2008). Continuous difficulties can lead to impairments such as poor readability, reduced speed, complaints of pain, tension and/or discomfort during writing, low self-esteem, less motivation for activities involving writing and a negative effect on the academic performance (Shen Lee, & Chen, 2012; Van Hartingsveldt et al., 2015).

THE DYSGRAPHIA

When an individual has an adequate intellectual level, he is given the necessary instructions for acquiring writing during elementary school, and is submitted to writing practice process during the academic training, and yet is unable to produce a comprehensive writing, this difficulty is denominated as dysgraphia (Rosenblum, Aloni, & Josman, 2010). According to the etymology of the word, dysgraphia derives from the concepts "dis" (deviation) + "spelling" (writing), that is, "a functional type disorder which affects the writing quality of the subject, regarding tracing or spelling" (Torres & Fernández, 2001, p. 127).

According to the DSM-5 (American Psychiatric Association [APA], 2013), a schoolchild with "specific learning disability with written expression deficiency" (coded 315.2 (F81.81)) presents disgraphy, when:

- he presents difficulty in relation to written expression, persisting for at least 6 months, despite the intervention sessions.
- has lower performance in writing skills than expected for the chronological age, related to readability (quality of letter formation, alignment and spacing of letters and words, and scaling of letters) and reduced speed (production rate)
- demonstrates difficulties in school or professional performance and daily living activities.
- difficulties are confirmed through full clinical evaluation and standardized performance measures.

Writing with impaired legibility can be characterized by changes in the quality of the letter formation, in the alignment and spacing of letters and words, in sizing of the letters and among others that impair the comprehension of the read material (Shen et al., 2012). Yet, the speed of writing refers to the accuracy and rate/quantity of letters and words written within a given period of time (Kim, Al Otaiba, Sidler, Greulich, & Puranik, 2014). They are directly linked to one another, since the schoolchildren need to write quickly, the quality/readability of the text may be affected; or if he writes more slowly, this may negatively affect writing productivity/quantity (Burger & McCluskey, 2011), since he may forget the ideas and intentions before writing them on the paper, impairing the textual production.

Studies demonstrate that boys and girls can present dysgraphia, in proportion of 2:1, respectively (Rubin & Henderson, 1982), schoolchildren with and without learning difficulties, with learning disorder, with dyslexia, Attention Deficit Hyperactivity Disorder (ADHD) and with autism (Cardoso & Capellini, 2016; Sumner, Connelly, & Barnett, 2012).

Students that present learning difficulties, do not acquire adequate strategies and competences for the development of writing, and they also present low motivation to be engaged in writing tasks (Graham & Harris, 2009). Yet, schoolchildren, according to studies by Martlew (1992) and Sumner et al., (2012), they show writing production rate slower than students without learning difficulties.

Studies by Mayes, Calhoun and Crowell (2000), about schoolchildren with ADHD showed that 70% of them had deficiencies in written expression, displaying illegible handwriting and poor letter formation. However, regarding writing speed, it is possible to find studies reporting that children with ADHD write isolated letters faster (Langmaid, Papadopoulos, Johnson, Phillips, & Rinehart, 2012), and studies which found out that their overall writing speed is slower, when compared to students proficient in writing (Shen et al., 2012).

Autistic children have presented difficulties concerning readability (Kushki, Chau, & Anagnostou, 2011), as they are unable to maintain letter size, presenting macrography (Cartmill, Roger, & Ziviani, 2009; Hellinckx, Roeyers, & Van Waelvelde, 2013). And as for students with ADHD, autistic writing speed is still a conflicting finding, since in the study by Hellinckx et al., (2013), it was slower when compared to proficient writers, but in the study by Cartmill et al., (2009), there was no significant difference between these groups.

THE HANDWRITING RESEARCH IN THE WORLD

Currently, in Brazil, there are few studies and evaluation tools with standardized performance measures which aim to investigate the quality and speed of manual writing, differently from other countries around the world, as observed in the Table below (Table 1), showing that it is possible to identify studies since 1910, and instruments since the 1980s.

Table 1. Survey in the international literature on how to evaluate writing

Authors	Evaluation	How	Instrument
Berninger et al., 1992, 1997.; Graham, Weintraub, 1996; Medwell, Wray, 2014	Legibility and speed	Write the alphabet and copy a pangram phrase in a certain time;	No
Alamargot, Morin, 2015	Legibility and speed	Write the alphabet; Write your first and last name	No
Gerth et al., 2016	legibility	Write the first name; copy a short 10x sentence	No
Lewis, Lewis, 1964	legibility	copy letters of the alphabet	No
Ritchey, 2008	legibility	Write letters by dictation	No
Graham, Weintraub, Berninger, 2001	legibility	Write letters seeking in memory	No
Puranik, Petscher, Lonigan, 2013	legibility	Write randomly dictated letters of the alphabet	No
Klein et al., 2011	legibility	Copy tasks, free writing by memory; written by dictation	No
Thorndike, 1910	legibility	Free writing	No
Ayres, 1912	Legibility and speed	Spontaneous writing; calculated the time that judges took to perform the manuscript reading	No
Collins et al., 1980; Helwing et al., 1976; Jones, Trap, Cooper, 1977	legibility	The sample of elaborate writing was arranged below a transparency, and the examiner/judge compared each letter of the written passage with the letters of transparency, by means of topographical characteristics	Yes - Transparent overlays
Rubin, Henderson, 1982	Legibility and speed	Copy a paragraph of 57 words on paper without lines in a period of five minutes. Writing speed was calculated as the number of letters written per minute.	Yes - Rubin and Henderson Scale
Hamstra-Bletz, De Bie, Den Brinker, 1987	Legibility and speed	Copy a standard text in five minutes or at least five lines if the child is a very slow writer. The speed is determined by counting the number of letters (including corrected letters) written in 5 minutes	Yes - The Concise Assessment Method for Children's Handwriting – BHK

Table 1. (Continued)

Authors	Evaluation	How	Instrument
Amundson, 1995	Legibility and speed	Write the memory alphabet using uppercase and lowercase letters, write memory numbers (1-12), dictation of both non-words and numbers, and sentence composition, with a test of 15 to 25 minutes.	Yes - The Evaluation Tool of Children's Handwriting-Manuscript - ETCH-M
Erez, Parush, 1999	Legibility and speed	Write all the letters of the Hebrew alphabet and 30 words/107 letters. Writing speed is measured by the number of letters produced during the first minute.	Yes - The Hebrew Handwriting Evaluation
Barnett et al., 2007	Legibility and speed	Copy of a sentence, memory alphabet writing, a percepto-viso-motor activity, and thematic writing. Each activity with a certain time.	Yes - Detailed Assessment of Speed of Handwriting – DASH
Reisman, 1999	legibility	Copy of a pangram sentence.	Yes - Minnesota Handwriting Assessment - MHA
Pollock et al., 2009	Legibility and speed	Write full name, numbers from 1 to 10, school name, alphabet, teacher's name, phone number, near and far copy, dictation and textual writing. Speed is calculated by number of letters/second in each task.	Yes - Handwriting Assessment Protocol

Observing the studies, it becomes possible to notice that, in general, manual writing is evaluated by means of copy, dictation and spontaneous writing (it can be the alphabet, phrases, texts, proper names or numbers). This analysis is performed either by an overall readability assessment (possible or not to understand what was written) and sometimes by different topographic characteristics, such as: letter size, letter shape, spaces between letters and words, line straightness writing, erasures, and so on. The writing speed is calculated in the publications, by letters/seconds, by words/seconds, by the time the writer performs the activity or by the time that the evaluator takes to read the written material.

Nevertheless, regardless of the instrument or methodology the evaluator will use to investigate handwriting, some considerations must be taken into account, so that erroneous requirements and comparisons do not lead to a false diagnosis. As follows:

- *Gender of the students evaluated*: according to an international study (Williams & Larkin, 2012), girls outnumber boys in speed and quality of writing and textual composition.
- *Age and schooling*: coordinated movements of writing improve with age and schooling, and consequently writing speed also increases (Sovik, 1993).
- *The writing request*: the type of text required also influences the speed, due to the cognitive demand that each task requires (Graham & Weintraub, 1996), thus, writing a self-generated text, for example, is more demanding than a copied text.
- *The instruction offered*: Depending on the instruction given to the student evaluated, such as "writing as fast as possible" or "writing trying to do your best," the writing pattern may be altered, favoring or impairing readability.
- *Ergonomic factors*: Attention should be paid to the pencil posture and handling during writing, as they can be modified throughout a writing task (Rosenblum, Goldstand, & Parush, 2006), reducing readability, pain, and fatigue in the upper limbs (Almeida, Sorensen, Magna, Cruz, & Ferrigno, 2013).
- *Investigation of other skills*: It becomes necessary to investigate perceptual-motor skills and fine motor skills as they are essential for handwriting (Thomassen & Teulings, 1983) and can help students to distinguish graphic forms, make possible corrections and form letters accurately (Tseng & Chow, 2000).

FINAL CONSIDERATIONS

This chapter was developed regarding the importance of manual writing nowadays, the consequences that a deficit in the development of this ability can cause to a student, and the difficulties in finding Brazilian studies concerning this subject. Whereas, despite the increased use of technology, with people using more electronic devices, such as mobile phones, smartphones and tablets to communicate, mastering writing skills still constitutes an important goal for school-aged-children (McCarney et al., 2013), and consequently deserves more attention from education and health professionals.

Acknowledgments

We are grateful to Capes (Coordination for the Improvement of Higher Education Personnel) for the PhD scholarship granted to the first author.

References

Ahmed, M., Rasool, A. G., Afzal, H., & Siddiqi I. (2017). Improving handwriting based gender classification using ensemble classifiers. *Expert Systems with Applications, 85* (1), 158-168. Accessed at: https://doi.org/10.1016/j.eswa.2017.05.033.

Almeida, P. H. T. Q., Sorensen, C. B. S., Magna L. A., Cruz D. M. C., & Ferrigno I. S. V. (2013). Avaliação da escrita através da fotogrametria – Estudo da preensão trípode dinâmica. *Revista de Terapia Ocupacional da Universidade de São Paulo* [Evaluation of writing through photogrammetry - Study of dynamic tripod hold. *Occupational Therapy Journal of the University of São Paulo*], *24* (1), 38-47.

American Psychiatric Association (2013). *Diagnostic and Statistical Manual of Mental Health Disorders*. 5th Edition. Arlington, VA: American Psychiatric Publishing.

Brazil. (2007). *Programa de Apoio a Leitura e Escrita - PRALER*. Brasília, DF: Ministério da Educação (MEC) e Secretaria de Educação Básica (SEB) [*Support Program for Reading and Writing - PRALER*. Brasília,

DF: Ministry of Education (MEC) and Secretariat of Basic Education (SEB)].

Burger, D. K., & McCluskey, A. (2011). Australian norms for handwriting speed in healthy adults aged 60–99 years. *Australian Occupational Therapy Journal, 58*, 355–363. doi: 10.1111/j.1440-1630.2011.00955.x.

Cardoso, M. H., & Capellini, S. A. (2016). Identificação e caracterização da disgrafia em escolares com dificuldades e transtornos de aprendizagem. *Distúrbios da Comunicação* [Identification and characterization of dysgraphia in schoolchildren with learning difficulties and disorders. *Communication Disorders, 28* (1), 27-37. Accessed at: <https://revistas.pucsp.br/index.php/dic/article/view/23948/19268>. Accessed on: 23 jul 2017.

Cartmill, L., Roger, S., & Ziviani, J. (2009). Handwriting of eight-year-old children with Autism Spectrum Disorder: An exploration. *Journal of Occupational Therapy, Schools and Early Intervention, 2* (2), 103–118. <http://dx.doi.org/10.1080/19411240903146426>. Accessed on: 19 out. 2016.

Chang, S. H., & Yu, N. Y. (2013). Handwriting movement analyses comparing first and second graders with normal or dysgraphic characteristics. *Research in Developmental Disabilities, 34* (9), 2433-2441. DOI: 10.1016/j.ridd.2013.02.028.

Duiser, I., Van Der Kamp, J., Ledebt, A., & Savelsbergh, G. (2014). Relationship between the quality of children's handwriting and the Beery Buktenica developmental test of visuomotor integration after one year of writing tuition. *Australian Occupational Therapy Journal, 61*, 76–82. http://dx.doi.org/10.1111/1440-1630.12064.

Graham, S., & Harris, K. R. (2009). Almost 30 years of writing research: making sense of it all with the wrath of khan. *Learning Disabilities Research & Practice*, 24, 58–68. doi: 10.1111/j.1540-5826.2009.01277.x.

Graham, S., & Weintraub, N. (1996). A review of handwriting research: progress and prospects from 1980 to 1994. *Educational Psychology Review*, 8, 7–88. doi:10.1007/BF01761831.

Hellinckx, T., Roeyers, H., & Van Waelvelde, H. (2013). Predictors of handwriting in children with Autism Spectrum Disorder. *Research in Autism Spectrum Disorders, 7* (1), 176—186. Accessed at: <http://dx.doi.org/10.1016/j.rasd.2012.08.009>. Accessed on: 20 out. 2016.

Kim, Y. S., Al Otaiba, S., & Wanzek, J. (2015). Kindergarten predictors of third grade writing. *Learning and Individual Differences, 37*, 27–37. doi:10.1016/j.lindif.2014.11.009.

Kim, Y. S., Al Otaiba, S., Sidler, J. F., Greulich, L., & Puranik, C. (2014). Evaluating the dimensionality of first grade written composition. *Journal of Speech, Language, and Hearing Research*, 57, 199–211. doi:10.1044/1092-4388.

Kushki, A., Chau, T., & Anagnostou, E. (2011). Handwriting difficulties in children with autism spectrum disorders: A scoping review. *Journal of Autism & Developmental Disorders, 41* (12), 1706–1716. Accessed at: <http://dx.doi.org/10.1007/s10803-011-1206-0>. Accessed on: 20 out. 2016.

Langmaid, R., Papadopoulos, N., Johnson, B., Phillips, J., & Rinehart, N. (2014). Handwriting in children with attention deficit hyperactivity disorder. *Journal of Attention Disorders, 18*, 504-510. doi:10.1177/1087054711434154.

Martlew, M. (1992). Handwriting and spelling: Dyslexic children's abilities compared with children of the same chronological age and younger children of the same spelling level. *British Journal of Educational Psychology, 62*, 375–390.

Mayes, S., Calhoun, S., & Crowell, E. (2000). Learning disabilities and ADHD: overlapping spectrum disorders. *Journal of Learning Disabilities, 33*, 417–424. doi: 10.1177/002221940003300502.

McCarney, D., Peters, L., Jackson, S., Thomas, M., & Kirby, A. (2013). Does poor handwriting conceal literacy potential in primary school children? *International Journal of Disability, Development and Education, 60*, 105-118. DOI: 10.1080/1034912X.2013.786561.

Medwell, J., & Wray, D. (2008). Handwriting – A forgotten language skill? *Language and Education, 22*, 34-47.

Miranda A. R. M. (2012). *Reflexões sobre a fonologia e a aquisição da linguagem oral e escrita* [*Reflections on phonology and the acquisition of oral and written language*]. Juiz de Fora, MG: Veredas Online – Especial. ISSN: 1982-2243.

Overvelde, A., & Hulstijn, W. (2011). Handwriting development in grade 2 and grade 3 primary school children with normal, at risk, or dysgraphic characteristics. *Research in Developmental Disabilities, 32* (2), 540–548. doi: 10.1016/j.ridd.2010.12.027.

Planton, S., Jucla, M., Roux, F. E., & Demonet J. F. (2013). The "handwriting brain": A meta-analysis of neuroimaging studies of motor versus orthographic processes. *Cortex, 49* (10), 2772-87. doi: 10.1016/j.cortex.2013.05.011.

Rosenblum, S., Aloni, T., & Josman, E. N. (2010). Relationships between handwriting performance and organizational abilities among children with and without dysgraphia: A preliminary study. *Research in Developmental Disabilities, 31*, 502-–509.

Rosenblum, S., Goldstand, S., & Parush, S. (2006). Relationships among biomechanical ergonomic factors, handwriting product quality, handwriting efficiency, and computerized handwriting process measures in children with and without handwriting difficulties. *American Journal of Occupational Therapy. 60* (1), 28-–39.

Rubin, N., & Henderson, S. E. (1982). Two sides of the same coin: Variation in teaching methods and failure to learn to write. *Special Education: Forward Trends, 9*, 17-24.

Sampaio, M. N., & Cardoso, M. H. (2015). A produção textual e a interferência da legibilidade e velocidade da escrita [The textual production and the interference of readability and speed of writing]. In Andrade, O. V. C. A., Okuda, P. M. M., & Capellini, S. A. (Orgs.) *Tópicos em Transtornos de aprendizagem* [*Topics in Learning Disorders*] (vol. 4, pp 73-88), Marília, SP: Fundepe, Cultura Acadêmica.

Schickedanz, J. A. (1999). *Much more than the ABCs: The early stages of reading and writing.* Washington, DC: National Association for the Education of Young Children.

Shen, I. H., Lee, T. Y., & Chen, C-L. (2012). Handwriting performance and underlying factors in children with Attention Deficit Hyperactivity Disorder. *Research in Developmental Disabilities, 33*, 1301–1309. Accessed at: <http://dx.doi.org/10.1016/j.ridd.2012.02.010>. Accessed on: 20 out. 2016.

Simonnet, D., Anquetil, E., & Bouillon, M. (2017). Multi-criteria handwriting quality analysis with online fuzzy models. *Pattern Recognition, 69,* 310-324. Accessed at https://doi.org/10.1016/j.patcog.2017.04.003.

Sovik, N. (1993). Development of children's writing performance: Some educational implications. In Kalverboer, A. F., Hopkins, B., & Geuze, R. (Eds.). *Motor development in early and later childhood: Longitudinal approaches.* (pp. 229-246). New York: Cambridge University Press.

Stevenson, N., & Just, C. (2014). In early education, why teach handwriting before keyboarding? *Early Childhood Education Journal, 42*, 49-56.

Sumner, E., Connelly, V., & Barnett, A. (2012). Children with dyslexia are slow writers because they pause more often and not because they are slow at handwriting execution. *Reading & Writing, 26* (6), 991-1008. Accessed at http://dx.doi.org/10.1007/s11145-012-9403-6.

Thomassen, J. W. M., & Teulings, H. M. (1983). The development of handwriting. In Martlew, M. (Ed.). *The psychology of written language: develop.*

Torres, R. M., & Fernández, P. F. (2001). *Dislexia, disortografia e disgrafia* [*Dyslexia, dysortography and dysgraphia*]. Lisboa: McGraw-Hill.

Tseng, M., & Chow, S. (2000). Perceptual-motor function of school-age children with slow handwriting speed. *American Journal of Occupational Therapy, 54*, 83–88.

Van Hartingsveldt, M. J., Cup E. H. C., Hendriks, J. C. M., Vries, L., Groot, I. J. M., & Nijhuis-Van Der Sanden, M. W. G. (2015). Predictive validity of kindergarten assessments on handwriting readiness. *Research in Developmental Disabilities, 36*, 114–124. DOI: 10.1016/j.ridd.2014.08.014.

Vinci-Booher, S., James, T. W., & James, K. H. (2016). Visual-motor functional connectivity in preschool children emerges after handwriting experience. *Trends in Neuroscience and Education, 5* (3), 107-120. Accessed at https://doi.org/10.1016/j.tine.2016.07.006.

Wertzner, H. F. (1995). Estudos da aquisição do sistema fonológico: o uso de processos fonológicos em crianças de três a seta anos. *Pró-fono: Revista de Atualização Cientifica* [Studies of the acquisition of the phonological system: the use of phonological processes in children from three to years arrow. *Pro-phone: Scientific Update Magazine*], *7*, (1), 21-26.

Whitehurst, G. J., & Lonigan C. J. (1998). Child development and emergent literacy. *Child Development, 69* (3), 848–872. Accessed at https://www.ncbi.nlm.nih.gov/pubmed/9680688.

Williams, G. J., & Larkin, R. F. (2012). Narrative writing, reading and cognitive processes in middle childhood: what are the links? *Learning and Individual Differences, 28*, 142-150. DOI: 10.1016/j.lindif. 2012.08.003.

In: Handwriting and Dysgrafia
Editors: M. Herrera Cardoso et al.
ISBN: 978-1-53613-805-4

Chapter 2

TRANSCULTURAL ADAPTATION OF THE HERE'S HOW I WRITE (HHIW) ASSESSMENT TOOL FOR BRAZILIAN CHILDREN

Juliana Flores Mendonça Alves[1,*], Adriana Maria Valladão Novais Van Petten[2], Ana Amélia Cardoso[2] and Lívia de Castro Magalhães[2]

[1]Laboratory of Studies on Learning Disorders (LETRA), HC/Universidade Federal de Minas Gerais, UFMG, Belo Horizonte, Minas Gerais, Brazil

[2]Department of Occupational Therapy, Universidade Federal de Minas Gerais UFMG, Belo Horizonte, Minas Gerais, Brazil

---

* Corresponding Author/Collaborator of the Laboratory of Studies on Learning Disorders (LETRA), jufloresto@gmail.com

ABSTRACT

Handwriting is an important tool for children in the process of literacy and school learning. Inadequate handwriting development, with slowness or illegibility, has a negative effect on school performance, which makes it important to identify handwriting difficulties as early as possible. Professionals working with school-aged children need valid and reliable instruments to assess and interpret handwriting problems, which would also facilitate the establishment of intervention programs and monitoring of their effects. Moreover, valid assessment tools are also essential for research. The Here's How I Write (HHIW) is a new, client-centered assessment tool that uses a self-evaluation questionnaire to include both the student and the teacher's perspective. Considering that the HHIW gives a view of several components of handwriting, according to the perspective of the student and the teacher, and that in Brazil we still do not have validated and accessible resources for handwriting evaluation, transcultural adaptation was done and the validity of the HHIW for Brazilian children was investigated. The translation process followed international recommendations for transcultural translation and adaptation of health-related questionnaires, following the stages of double translation, elaboration of a translated unified version, back-translation, synthesis with preparation of the pre-final version, pre-test and, finally, the use of the HHIW-Brazil in a target sample to analyze its psychometric properties. HHIW-Brazil was applied to 60 children aged 8 to 10 years old from public and private schools (30 good handwriters and 30 poor handwriters) and their teachers. The results support the reliability and validity of the HHIW-Brazil as well as its clinical utility, as it is a resource of rapid application and was well accepted by Brazilian children and teachers. The publication of the HHIW-Brazil is recommended as it seems useful for clinical use and research. More studies are required to fully validate the translated instrument.

Keywords: handwriting, evaluation, cross-cultural adaptation, client-centered practice

INTRODUCTION

Handwriting is one of the most important tools for human communication (Wallen, Duff, Goyen, & Froude, 2013), a tool that is used to record information, complete tasks, perform tests and interact with other people (Yinon & Weintraub, 2000; Peverly, 2006). It is also an important skill in the literacy and school learning processes (Falk, Tam, Schwellnus & Chau, 2010) because it is a way for children to express their learning, creativity, and knowledge (Wallen et al., 2013).

It is estimated that 30% to 60% of a child's day at school is occupied with fine motor activities (McHale & Cermak, 1992), and a significant period of this time is dedicated to handwriting (Feder & Majnemer, 2007). Handwriting is a complex task that involves not only fine motor coordination, but also factors such as grip type and strength, and pencil and body positioning, besides performance skills such as integrity of the visuomotor coordination, perceptual skills, motor planning, and cognition (Amundson, 2005). Other important aspects of handwriting development are interest and motivation (Rosenblum, Weiss, & Parush, 2003). It is expected that between the ages of 10 and 12 years these factors and performance skills are already developed, however, some children continue to have handwriting difficulties (Rueckriegel et al., 2008).

Handwriting difficulties impact on academic performance (Graham, Harris & Fink, 2000; Jones & Christensen, 1999) and can affect many areas of life, with consequent loss of self-confidence, reduction in career opportunities, and even difficulties in personal relationships (Sassoon, 1997). Depending on the sample and type of instrument used to evaluate the written production (i.e., letter formation, not spelling and grammatical issues), the prevalence of handwriting difficulties among school-aged children varies from 10% to 34% (Rubin, Henderson, Smits-Engelsman et al., 2001).

In general, handwriting problems are characterized by too large or too small strokes, or even both, fluctuation in letter size and in the positioning on the line, excessively slow or fast writing rhythm, letters too spread out, overlapping or illegible, in addition to inadequate body posture (Coelho, 2013). Facing the requirements of attention and the effort required to draw the letters, the child may forget what he or she wanted to write, leaving out letters or words, producing illegible handwriting, and writing at low speed, the main handwriting problems observed in children at school (Rosenblum,

Weiss, & Parush, 2003). Children with handwriting problems often experience anxiety and frustration when are asked to complete homework, register events on an agenda, or write an essay (Rosenblum, Weiss & Parush, 2004).

Although the need to invest in handwriting is currently being questioned as technological resources can be used to replace it, there is evidence that handwriting plays an important role in the organization of brain circuits, which facilitates the development of reading and is associated with various aspects of academic success (James & Engelhardt, 2012; Dinehart, 2014). Moreover, as the use of technological resources at home and classroom is not yet a reality for most children, especially in Brazil, handwriting continues to be an important skill of daily life that deserves attention from educators and health professionals (Feder & Majnemer, 2007).

Besides teachers, other professionals working in the school system, such as occupational therapists, play an important role in the evaluation and development of programs aimed at improving the handwriting quality (Schneck & Amundson, 2010). These professionals need valid and reliable instruments to assess and interpret handwriting problems, establish intervention programs, monitor the effects of the intervention, and conduct research to get a better understanding of the handwriting mechanisms (Feder, Majnemer & Synnes, 2000).

There are several instruments for evaluating handwriting. They can be seen in Table 1, which presents the tests most cited in the literature: Evaluation Tool of Children's Handwriting (ETCH) (Amundson, 1995), Minnesota Handwriting Assessment (MHA) (Reisman, 1999), Concise Assessment Method for Children's Handwriting (BHK) (Hamstra-Beltz, Bie & Brinker, 1987), Test of Handwriting Skills (Gardner, 1998); Children's Handwriting Evaluation System (CHES) (Phelps, Stemple & Speck, 1984), Detailed Assessment of Speed of Handwriting (DASH) (Barnett, Henderson, Scheib & Schultz, 2007) and Here's How I Write (HHIW) (Goldstand, Gervir, Cermak, & Bissell, 2013). Each test covers one or more handwriting components - quality, readability, speed, letter formation, alignment, size, and spacing of writing. As shown in Table 1, the most complete instrument is the HHIW, as it encompasses all evaluated components from the other instruments and, as described below, incorporates a self-evaluation component as a means to promote the child's interest and motivation to write.

Table 1. Components evaluated by the main instruments for assessing the quality and readability of handwriting

	BHK	CHES	DASH	ETCH	MAH	THS	HHIW
Readability		X		X	X	X	X
Speed		X	X	X			X
Form					X		X
Alignment					X		X
Size					X		X
Spacing					X		X
Quality	X				X		X

Note: BHK = Concise Evaluation Scale for Children's Handwriting, CHES = Children`s Handwriting Evaluation System, DASH = Detailed Assessment of Speed of Handwriting, ETCH Evaluation Tool of Children´s Handwriting, MHA= Minnesota Handwriting Assessment, THS Test of Handwriting Skills, HHIW = Here's How I Write.

Here's How I Write

The HHIW is a recent instrument (Goldstand, Gervir, Cermak, & Bissell, 2013) that differs from others as it proposes a self-evaluation of handwriting, through an interview based questionnaire directed to the student. It also involves the teacher, who answers a questionnaire with the same questions. was created according to the principles of the client-centered practice, one of the pillars of current occupational therapy (AOTA, 2014), which advocates that therapists should seek to involve the child in the process of assessment and intervention, using strategies that facilitate self-assessment and enable collaboration in the definition of treatment goals (Amundson, 2005). There is evidence that when children have the opportunity to exercise control over their work and to set their own goals, there is greater involvement in the evaluation process and greater collaboration during therapy (Graham, Harris & McKeown, 2013). In addition, the child becomes more self-determined and therefore more motivated to learn, achieving better outcomes in the treatment goals (Missiuna, Pollack & Law, 2004; Ryan & Deci, 2000). Therefore, self-assessment plays a fundamental role in promoting learning, because of its motivating effect (Toglia, 2011).

HHIW was created by occupational therapists from Israel and the United States. Its original version was published in Hebrew (Goldstand & Gevir, 2006, 2009) and then translated into English (Goldstand, Gervir, Cermak, & Bissell, 2013). The psychometric qualities of the child and teacher questionnaires were investigated in both countries, supporting the reliability and validity of the instrument.

As described by the authors (Goldstand, Gervir, Cermak, & Bissell, 2013), the original questionnaire, when applied to Israeli children, had high internal consistency ($\alpha = 0.884$) and moderate test-retest reliability ($r = 0.614$) with children without difficulty in handwriting. In children with poor handwriting, a significant correlation was found between the HHIW score and a dysgraphia test ($r = 0.63$) and between the child and teacher scores ($r = 0.71$) on the HHIW. The agreement between the responses of the children and the teachers was 70-88%.

In the North American version, Cermak and Bissell (2014) found a significant difference between the results of children with poor and good handwriting ($p < 0.001$) and a moderate correlation between the children's and teachers' total scores ($r = 0, 62$). When comparing only the scores of children with good handwriting and the teacher a significant difference ($p < 0,0001$) was found, however, in the group with poor handwriting, the difference was not significant ($p = 0.11$) (Cermak & Bissell et al., 2014). These studies indicate that HHIW is a valid and reliable instrument to help children identify their handwriting difficulties.

The HHIW is easy to use and understand since the children's questionnaire was transformed into pictorial cards, which illustrate the skills related to handwriting. There are 25 pictorial cards and one is an example to help the child understand how the self-evaluation process works. In all cards, the front and back are illustrated with figures and sentences in pairs, for the child to identify if their performance is good (front) or poor (verse) in specific components of the handwriting.

The HHIW involves the child through the process of choosing the figures with which he/she best identifies. For each pair, the child points out which side best expresses his/her performance and classifies it as "sometimes" or "always." That also helps in identifying the difficulties, which can be transformed into intervention objectives and then re-evaluated, as a means to improve handwriting.

The HHIW cards are divided into three categories: (1) two items involving the child's feelings in relation to handwriting (e.g., "I like to write," "I feel I write well"), (2) three items related to physical factors, including body posture and stabilizing the page with the non-writing hand (e.g., "I sit right in my chair"), and (3) 19 items with specific figures that illustrate writing performance (for example, "I write over the line"). The teacher´s questionnaire has the same items pictured in the cards, which allows a comparison between the perspective of the child and the teacher's. Based on the child's and teacher's scores, the items or areas of greatest difficulty are identified, which in discussion with the child, are transformed into goals/aims to be worked in a certain period of time, followed by re-evaluation.

The HHIW helps children and teachers in identifying handwriting problems, and then, in partnership with the therapist, seeking solutions to improve the performance (Goldstand, Gervir, Cermak, & Bissell, 2013). Due to the focus on the child's self-assessment and collaboration in the definition of treatment goals, the instrument does not present normative scores. Thus, HHIW is not a test, but it contributes to identify areas of greater difficulty, which requires specific evaluation, and engagement of the child, teacher and therapist in the definition of intervention objectives consistent with the reality of the classroom.

The HHIW manual also includes ideas for improving performance on specific items, as each card comes with intervention suggestions, which can be applied both at school and at home. From the cards in which the child identifies his/her performance as poor, the therapist, in partnership with the teacher and the child, develops intervention strategies. For example, when the child points to the "I do not like writing," the therapist and teacher can: try to integrate the child's interests into handwriting activities (e.g., if the child likes soccer, he or she can copy texts related to this theme); evaluate the importance of each handwriting exercise and eliminate the unnecessary ones; talk about the importance of handwriting in the child's life and give positive reinforcement during handwriting activities.

If the child chooses the "I cannot read and understand what I write," the therapist can evaluate the components needed for handwriting (e.g., visual perception, visual-motor coordination) and, in partnership with the child, create fun activities to develop these components, as well as practice handwriting. Or, when the child indicates by the card "I do not sit upright in my chair," the therapist should evaluate ergonomic aspects of the student's desk and chair for proper accommodation or necessary adaptations. For good handwriting performance, the child should sit comfortably with the hip and knees at a 90-degree angle, their feet should be resting on the floor, and the elbows leaning forward on the table. Another strategy would be to guide the teacher to provide sensory breaks during the class, incorporating exercises such as: standing and stretching the body, shaking hands and arms, pushing the wall with arms outstretched, joining the palms of the hands in front of the chest and breathing deep three times. For each card, there are several suggestions for intervention and adaptations, which extends the use of the HHIW beyond just identifying areas of difficulty.

The decision to conduct the cross-cultural adaptation and analysis of the validity of the HHIW for the Brazilian children was based on the importance of evaluating handwriting at school age and the absence of validated instruments, with available manuals and protocols, for clinical use and research in Brazil. We also considered the characteristics of HHIW, an instrument that incorporates both evaluation and intervention aspects. For the translation and adaptation of the HHIW-US version to Brazil, authorization was first requested from the author, Dr. Sharon

Cermak, and the publisher, who approved the translation for research purposes. The translation process followed the six stages recommended by Beaton, Bombardier, Guillemin & Ferraz, (2000) for cross-cultural adaptation of health related questionnaires, as described in Figure 1, resulting in the HHIW-Brazil (Alves, 2015).

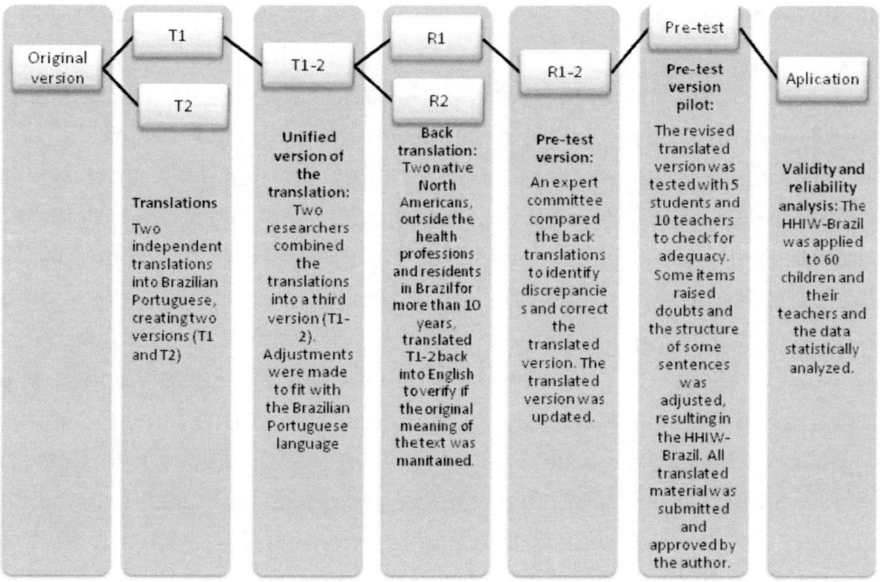

Figure 1. Steps in the process of cross-cultural adaptation of the HHIW (Alves, 2015, p. 22).

During the translation, in order to facilitate comprehension by the teachers and students, some modifications were made so that the items' statements were more consistent with the language used in the schools, but without changing the original meaning of each item. Some items have been modified to adjust for the semantic equivalence criterion, with substitution of words ("We write within the margins of the page/We do not write within the margins of the page" for "I write inside the edges of the sheet/ I do not write inside the edges of the sheet"), omission of words ("My letters are about the same size" by the phrase "My letters are the same size") and addition of words ("Write well/Do not write well" by the phrase "Write well (readable)/Do not write well (unreadable)"). In the pre-test phase, the researchers discussed items that raised doubts among either the teachers or children and made minor adjustments until the final version was considered adapted to the Brazilian school context (Alves, 2015).

After the translation, in order to confirm reliability and validity, the HHIW-Brazil was applied to 60 children aged 8 to 10 years (30 with good handwriting and 30 with poor handwriting), from public and private schools, matched by age, gender and social class (Alves, 2015). The teachers and children answered the translated questionnaire. Both children and teachers responded to the questionnaires twice, within a 15-day interval, to verify the test-retest reliability of the translated version.

The interview with the child took about 15 minutes, and both the children and the teachers liked the instrument. The teachers considered the questionnaire quite complete, with only a few reports of uncertainty to score specific questions about the performance of some children, such as where the letter begins on the line and signs of fatigue. The children were enthusiastic about the opportunity to evaluate their own handwriting. HHIW-Brazil presented excellent test and retest reliability indexes for both the teacher and child questionnaires (ICC = 0.930, 0.964, respectively), demonstrating that the items are clear, easy to understand, and that students and teachers can respond in a reliable way. HHIW was effective in differentiating the quality of handwriting in children with good and poor handwriting, because there were significant difference between the groups, both in the total self-assessment score of the child and in the teachers' evaluation ($p = 0.0001$) as well as in the three categories or subgroups of items of the questionnaires. The results suggested that Brazilian children aged 8 to 10 years are able to evaluate their own performance in handwriting tasks.

Of the 24 questions of the instrument, in only seven (29%) there was no statistically significant agreement between the student and teacher scores However, the agreement was high for the total score of the questionnaires (ICC = 0.749, $p = 0.0001$). This indicates that children and teachers share perceptions about the areas of difficulty, and in items where there was disagreement, the differences were more related to the perception of the degree of difficulty (score 1 or 2) than to opposing visions concerning the quality of the performance on the item.

The process of cross-cultural adaptation was completed and the HHIW-Brazil was well evaluated by children and teachers. Reliability and validity data suggest that the instrument retained the original psychometric properties when used with Brazilian children, constituting an innovative resource to subsidize intervention of the occupational therapist and other professionals who work in schools. The next step in making the HHIW-Brazil feasible is to publish the manual with the assessment protocols in Portuguese, which depends on negotiation with the publisher. However, as the questionnaire was translated in Belo Horizonte, Minas Gerais, seeking to use language that is closer to the one spoken in the local school context, the translation of the cards and teacher questionnaire may need adjustments to be used in other regions of the country, an issue that should be investigated in future studies.

CONCLUSION

The HHIW is an instrument that contributes to client-centered practice and it adjusts easily into the clinical practice of the Brazilian occupational therapist. The questionnaire stands out because it provides information on a greater number of handwriting components and, at the same time, it motivates, instigates and involves the children through the cards, allowing them to express their perceptions about the quality of their own handwriting. The instrument includes the teacher's view, which tends to be consistent with that of the child, helping to target intervention goals to the demands of the classroom context.

The process of transcultural translation and adaptation was carefully conducted, resulting in an instrument that can be used both in research and in the practice of Brazilian professionals. The initial data support the reliability and validity of the HHIW-Brazil, but it is important to investigate whether the scores of the instrument are consistent with handwriting measures obtained with normative tests, validated for the

Brazilian children. It should also be investigated whether the self-evaluation, in fact, contributes to the child's greater engagement in the intervention, contributing to success in handwriting.

REFERENCES

Alves, J. F. M. (2015). *Adaptação transcultural e análise da validação do Here's How I Write: auto-avaliação da escrita.* [Transcultural adaptation and validation analysis of Here's How I Write: self-evaluation of writing.] Dissertação de mestrado. Programa de Pós Graduação em Ciências da Reabilitação, Universidade de Federal de Minas Gerais, Belo Horizonte.

American Occupational Therapy Association. (2014). *American Journal of Occupational Therapy,* 68(48) doi:10.5014/ajot.2014.682006.

Amundson, S. J. (1995). *Evaluation Tool of Children's Handwriting.* Homer, AK: O. T. Kids Inc.

Amundson, S. J. (2005). Prewriting and Handwriting Skill. In: Case-Smith, J. *Occupational Therapy for Children.* (5rd ed., pp.304-56). United States, Ed Evolve.

Barnett, A., Henderson, S. E., Scheib, B. & Schulz, J.. (2007). *Detailed* Assessment of Speed of Handwriting (DASH). London: Pearson.

Beaton, D. E., Bombardier, C., Guillemin, F. & Ferraz, M. B. (2000). Guidelines for the process of cross-cultural adaptation of self-report measures. *SPINE*, 25 (24), 3186-3191.

Cermak, S. A. & Bissell, J. (2014) Content and construct validity of Here's How I Write (HHIW): A Child's Self-Assessment and Goal Setting Tool. *American Journal of Occupational Therapy*, 68(3), 296-306. doi: 10.5014/ajot.2014.010637.

Coelho, D. T. (2013). *Dificuldades de Aprendizagem específicas: Dislexia, Disgrafia, Disortografia e Discalculia* [*Specific Learning Disabilities: Dyslexia, Dysgraphia, Disortography and Dyscalculia*]. Porto: Areal Editoras.

Dinehart, L. (2014). Handwriting in early childhood education: Current research and future implications. *Journal of Early Childhood Literacy*, 15(1), 1-22.

Falk, T., H, Tam, C., Schwellnus, H. & Chau, T. (2010). Grip force variability and its effects on children's handwriting legibility, form, and strokes. *Journal Biomedical Engineering,* 132(11): 114504. doi: 10.1115/1.4002611.

Feder, K., Majnemer, A. & Synnes, A. (2000). Handwriting: current trends in occupational therapy practice. *Canadian Journal Occupational Therapy,* 67(3), 197-204.

Feder, K. P. & Majnemer, A. (2007). Handwriting development, competency, and intervention. *Developmental Medicine and Child Neurology*, 49(4), 312-7.

Gardner, M. (1998). *THS: Test of Handwriting Skills.* Hydesville, CA: Psychological and Educational Publications.

Graham, S. K. R., Harris, B. & Fink, B. (2000). Is handwriting causally related to learning to write? Treatment of handwriting problems in beginning writers. *Journal of Educational Psychology*, 92(4), 620–33. http://dx.doi.org/10.1037/0022-0663.92.4.620.

Graham, S., Harris, K. R., & McKeown, D. (2013). The writing of students with learning disabilities, meta-analysis of self-regulated strategy development writing intervention studies, and future directions: Redux. In H. Swanson, K. R. Harris, & S. Graham (Eds.), *Handbook of learning disabilities* (2nd ed., pp. 405–438). New York: Guilford Press.

Goldstand, S. & Gevir, D. (2006, 2009) Research on the Hebrew Versuion. In: Goldstand, S., Gevir, D., Cermak, S., & Bissell, J. (2013). *Here's How I Write: A Child's Self-Assessment and Goal Setting Tool.* Framingham, MA: Therapro.

Goldstand, S., Gevir, D., Cermak, S., & Bissell, J. (2013). *Here's How I Write: A Child's Self-Assessment and Goal Setting Tool*. Framingham, MA: Therapro.

Hamstra-Beltz, L., Bie, D. J., & Brinker, D. B. (1987). *Concise evaluation scale for children's handwriting, BHK.* Lisse, Netherlands: Swets & Zeitlinger.

James, K. H. & Engelhardt, L. (2012). The effects of handwriting experience on functional brain development in pre-literate children, *Trends in Neuroscience and Education*, 1 (1), 32-42.

Jones, D. & Christensen, C. A. (1999). Relationship between automaticity in handwriting and student's ability to generate written text. *Journal of Educational Psychology* 91: 44-49.

Mchale, K. & Cermak, S. S. (1992). Fine motor activities in elementary school: Preliminary findings and provisional implications for children with fine motor problems. *American Journal of Occupational Therapy*, 46(10), 898-903.

Missiuna, C., Pollack, N., & Law, M. (2004). *The Perceived Efficacy and Goal Setting System*. Toronto, Ontario: Psychological Corporation.

Phelps, J., Stempel, L., & Speck, G. (1984). *Children's handwriting, evaluation scale*. Dallas, TX: Scottish Rite Hospital for Crippled Children.

Peverly, S. T. (2006). The importance of handwriting speed in adult writing, *Dev Neuropsychol.* 29(1), 197-216.

Reisman, J. (1999). *Minnesota Handwriting Assessment manual.* San Antonio, TX: Harcourt Assessment Inc.

Ryan, R. M., & Deci E. L. (2000). Intrinsic and Extrinsic Motivations: Classic Definitions and New Directions, *Contemporary Educational Psychology*, 25, 54–67.

Rosenblum, S., Weiss, P. L. & Parush, S. (2004) Handwriting evaluation for developmental dysgrafia: Process versus Product. *An Interdisciplinary Journal*. 17(5), 433-58.

Rosenblum, S., Weiss, S. P. L., & Parush, S. (2003). Product and process evaluation of handwriting difficulties: A review. *Educational Psychology Review,* 15, 41–81.

Rubin, N. & Henderson, S. E. (1982). Two sides of the same coin: Variation in teaching methods and failure to learn to write. *Special Education: Forward Trends* 9: 17- 24.

Rueckriegel, S. M. et al. (2008) Influence of age and movement complexity on kinematic hand movement parameters in childhood and adolescence. *International Journal Developmental Neuroscience*, 26(7), 655-663.

Sassoon, R. (1997). Dealing with adult handwriting problems. *Handwriting Review* 11: 69-74.

Schneck, C. & Amundson, S. (2010). Prewriting and writing. In J. Case-Smith & J. O'Brien (Eds.) *Occupational Therapy for Children. (6th ed)* (pp. 555-582). St. Louis: Mosby/Elsevier.

Toglia, J. (2011). Cognition, occupation, and participation across the life span. In Cermak, S. A., &, Bissell, J. (2014). Content and construct validity of Here's How I Write (HHIW): A Child's Self-Assessment and Goal Setting Tool. *American Journal Occupational Therapy*, 68(3), 296-306. doi: 10.5014/ajot.2014.010637.

Wallen, M., Duff, S., Goyen, T. & Froude, E. (2013). Respecting the evidence: Responsible assessment and effective intervention for children with handwriting difficulties. *Australian Occupational Therapy Journal,* 60 (5), 366–369. doi: 10.1111/1440-1630.12045.

Yinon, M., & Weintraub, N. (2000). Intervention programs for improving handwriting performance: A review. *Israel Journal of Occupational Therapy,* 9,17–35.

In: Handwriting and Dysgrafia
Editors: M. Herrera Cardoso et al.
ISBN: 978-1-53613-805-4

Chapter 3

ASSESSMENT OF THE HANDWRITING QUALITY: AN INSTRUMENT FOR THE BRAZILIAN EDUCATIONAL CONTEXT

Adriane Guzman Pasculli Milani[1,*], Cynthia Yukiko Hiraga[2] and Ana Maria Pellegrini[2]

[1]São Paulo State University "Júlio de Mesquita Filho" (UNESP), Graduate Program in Human Development and Technologies, Biosciences Institute, Campus of Rio Claro (Rio Claro), Brazil

[2]São Paulo State University "Júlio de Mesquita Filho" (UNESP), Biosciences Institute, Campus of Rio Claro (Rio Claro), Brazil

ABSTRACT

Handwriting is a complex skill exclusive to the human being. It is indispensable for the individual to integrate and adapt to our social environment. It is a complex skill that involves a combination of perceptual, motor, kinesthetic, and cognitive components. The assessment of handwriting is one of the challenges encountered by teachers who

* Corresponding Author Email: dripasculli@yahoo.com.br

work with the literacy process. This chapter presents the Minnesota Handwriting Assessment (MHA), an instrument developed by Judith Reisman and used in English speaking language countries, as a possible tool for assessing the quality of the handwriting in the Brazilian educational context. Such an instrument allows us to determine the quality of each child's handwriting objectively, as well as to evaluate the progress of these children and the class as a whole. The results per variable of the quality of the handwriting could provide teachers valuable information regarding the sensory-motor abilities involved in the production of the handwriting.

Keywords: handwriting, assessment, children

1. Introduction

Among a wide range of human productions is the handwriting, a relevant form of communication of human development. The handwriting is a complex activity that involves the integration of perceptual, motor, kinesthetic and cognitive components. For example, a text written by hand requires from the individual planning, grammatical skills, monitoring of the direction of the handwriting, motor coordination, among other capabilities. The handwriting is one of the activities that distinguishes the human being from other species, with significant social, cultural and scholarly-academic value. Handwriting is one of ways that humans record their thoughts, their emotions and a whole set of activities related to the acquisition of knowledge and social interaction (Tam, Ryan, Rigby, 2009). The development of handwriting begins with the first scribbles that become, over time, more intentional and more precise. The forms of the letters can be seen in the children's drawings, indicating initial learning of the handwriting (Feder & Majnemer, 2007).

The handwriting has a dimension that goes beyond the classroom because it is essential for the individual to integrate and adapt to the social environment. The acquisition of handwriting allows children to make use of it in different ways depending on the context, such as during play, communication, expression of thought, among others. An instrument of assessment for the handwriting should be included in the first years of academic learning. The acquisition of skill literacy not only involves the knowledge of letters, syllabus, and words but the production of good handwriting strokes. The acquisition of handwriting permits the individuals to fully explore the environment, communicate with other participants in any context, serve to various uses and functions inherent in a literate society build in a personal rhythm (Brito, 2007). Although nowadays the predominance of digital technologies in the many everyday activities, including children in school, handwriting has not become dispensable or obsolete.

Among different aspects of handwriting that can be analyzed, the present work limits to examine the production of handwriting stroke. Children in the literacy process are seeking to master the writing skill and also attempting to produce the alphabet letters of good quality. The little attention of pedagogical guidance to produce the letters and other factors associated with the literacy process may compromise the quality of handwriting strokes in general process of the child's schooling (Federer & Majnemer, 2007). In particular, children with learning disabilities may find more challenging to learn the handwriting strokes during the literacy process adequately. This may compromise communication and academic performance and, consequently, the child's emotional development (Rosemblum, Weiss & Parush, 2003).

In the process of handwriting acquisition, the child learns to identify and differentiate the pattern of strokes of the various letters of the alphabet from the model presented by the teacher on the blackboard. On the other hand, many children have difficulties in handwriting, with a poor pattern of strokes regarding form, legibility, alignment of letters and spacing between letters and words, which might likely affect their academic performance. Poor quality of handwriting, for example, may affect the reading of her/his writing, the development of reasoning for the text composition, the speed of handwriting. In general, a poor pattern of strokes of the letters ultimately may difficult to monitor the academic learning of the child.

The production of handwriting requires the user to hold either a pencil or pen, coordinate and control the movement of the fingers and wrist in a manner that the product of the handwriting might transmit the message or information to the reader (Rosemblum, Weiss & Parush, 2003). The act of handwriting always involves an appropriate hand contact with the pen and the pen with the support surface. The accuracy of form of the letter is a prerequisite for the legibility, and then the reader readily identifies the written letter to give a meaning to the word and the text as a whole. The excellent quality of the handwriting demands to memorize the layout of each letter simultaneously with the arrangement of the set of specific motor commands for the production of the letter (Bara & Gentaz, 2010). When the child does not fully incorporate the pattern of the letters of the alphabet by the child, the harmony of the set of the handwriting strokes for the letters composing each word may not be achieved.

From the motor point of view, a good quality of handwriting demands the individual to adjust muscular contractions of the fingers, wrist, and elbow, which requires an appropriate manipulation of the pencil. Handwriting requires fine and precise control of upper limb components, such as muscles, tendons, and joints along the hand, forearm, and arm (Latash, Danion, Scholz, Zatsiortsky & Schöner, 2003). Finger force control enables oscillatory movements to be performed efficiently, and the pencil grip is properly implemented, favoring the quality of handwriting (Schneck & Henderson, 1990; Tseng & Cermark, 1993). Latash et al. (2003) argue that the child's difficulty in adequately activating specific musculoskeletal structures for the ability of handwriting may be a determining factor for the poor handwriting pattern in the school setting.

2. The Acquisition of the Handwriting

The act of handwriting demands time for acquisition and learning. The acquisition begins when the child is still small and discovers objects, manipulating them first with palmar grip, with immature and primitive grips. The most common form of holding the pen or pencil according to literature is the dynamic tripod (Elliot & Connoly, 1984; Schneck & Henderson, 1990). For both children and adults, in this type of grip, the pencil is secured and controlled by the forefinger and thumb, gripped on the lateral distal surface of the third finger (Elliot & Connolly, 1984). However, according to Sodre (2000), in many cases, inefficient grips hinder the acquisition of the motor skills of handwriting that impacts on the quality of handwriting.

The child initiates the manipulation of the pencil around the age of two, using hand grips with crossed or supinated palmar grip that over time improves becoming more mature. At four years of age, the child already holds the pencil with the thumb, and two of the other fingers, such as the index finger and the middle extended, controlling the pen in such a way that he/she can copy a circle, draw a cross and sketch drawings of human forms and houses. From four to six years old, the child holds the pencil with the most proper grips, and also has transitional grips that need to be refined, such as the crossed thumb, quadruple and static tripod grips. These grips still present limitations on the joint dissociation of the fingers, not allowing a good quality of the handwriting (Sodré, 2000).

Approximately between six and seven years old, the child can reach maturity on the handwriting grip, presenting a pattern for support and manipulation of the pencil, with more efficient grips for handwriting, such as lateral tripod types and dynamic tripod. These types of grips allow joint dissociation of the phalanges and wrist, lower energy expenditure, and lower muscle strength, giving the child fun to draw and paint human forms, houses or objects with clarity. At this stage, the process of literacy and the acquisition of handwriting begins, with the emergence of the most proper grips for the progression of good handwriting (Sodré, 2000).

In summary, to produce handwriting, the individual needs to define the type and size of the letter, the space between words and lines, specify the trajectories of the displacement of the body segments in space. Furthermore, to specify the force in the vertical direction that determines the physical characteristics of the path (depth and width), the size of the displacements and the speed of trajectories according to constraints imposed by the environment and/or by the individual (Calvo, Pasculli, Hiraga, Del Masso & Pellegrini, 2014). Also, to adjust the body posture and the inclination of the paper to favor good handwriting. The handwriting grip is also a determining factor on the quality of the handwriting in the measure that plays a role on the production of the strokes and on the energy consumption for producing the traces resulting from the pressure of the pencil on the paper.

3. Handwriting in Public Educational Policies

The National Pact for Literacy on the Right Age (Brazil, 2013) "is a formal commitment made by the federal government, to Federal District, state and municipal governments to ensure that all children are literate until the age of eight, at the end of the 3rd year of Elementary School." In the context of literacy, not only the writing but the handwriting stroke should be dominated by students, including disabled children. The adherence to the Pact, the government institutions are responsible for: I. Literacy of all children in Portuguese and developing skills in the field of mathematics. II. To carry out annual universal assessments, applied by Inep, of the students of the 3rd year of Elementary School. III. It is up to the states to support the municipalities that have adhered to the actions of the Pact, for their effective implementation.

The actions of the Pact include an integrated set of programs, materials and curricular and pedagogical references to be provided by the Ministry of Education in which contribute to the literacy process, with the primary focus on the continuing education of literacy teachers. With the Pact, the literate child must master the alphabetical system of the handwriting, be able to read and write, with autonomy. It should be noted here that even with all the efforts of the Brazilian government and educational researchers to improve the teaching/learning process, what is observed in the classroom is not in line with what is proposed in the Pact. Also, the domain of the alphabetic system by the child must also include the facet relating to the production of handwriting strokes.

In general, in the elementary school students do not have the necessary primary skills that should be developed in children's education, specifically those related to handwriting. From the motor-sensory point of view, for example, the development of fine-finger coordination skills, as well as the development of visual-motor integration, should be part of the scheduling of school activities to strengthen sensorimotor patterns specifically for the production of the handwriting strokes.

Another point of debate in teaching practice, according to the teachers, concerns the proposal arguing for not making use of the demonstration to children of a correct pattern to produce the trajectory of each alphabet letters. Thus, freedom is given to the child to present his style and manner to produce his/he own handwriting strokes. The National Pact is concerned with the field of writing and reading. However, it does not refer to the quality of the handwriting strokes. Therefore, the quality of handwriting in Brazilian education is not considered a determining factor that could interfere with the literacy process.

4. The Assessment of Handwriting

The use of standardized tests to evaluate the quality of handwriting or the direct observation of teachers can facilitate the identification of handwriting performance standards. Such evaluation is relevant since the handwriting is the instrument that allows the assessment of the acquisition of knowledge. According to Racine, Majnemer, Shevell, and Snider (2008), a standardized, valid and reliable assessment instrument provides quantitative scores that enable the examiner to measure the progression of the individual throughout the acquisition and learning processes.

There is a lack in Brazil of assessment methods and instruments for the handwriting in the context of the school, which has motivated researchers to seek tools in other languages and cultures that could be used after adaptation and validation to the Brazilian context. According to Fuentes, Mostofsky, and Bastian (2009), the Minnesota Handwriting Assessment (Reisman, 1999) is an instrument for assessing handwriting whose results are close to reports of writing difficulties pointed out by children's teachers. Consequently, such an instrument can be seen as an easy-to-manage tool that can be incorporated into the procedures to be used by teachers in the process of literacy acquisition.

The MHA is an instrument of qualitative evaluation of the handwriting stroke in English which consists of copying a printed letter style sentence (the quick brown fox jumps over the lazy dog) involving all the letters of the English alphabet (i.e., pangram). The phrase containing all the letters of the alphabet for the Portuguese language – *um pequeno jabuti xereta viu dez cegonhas felizes* - in the stick letter style was used according to the adaptation already made by Calvo et al. (2014) and later validation by Pasculli (2014). The material to carry out this assessment included an A4 sheet containing the sentence to be copied and guidelines with standardized space for the execution of the copy of the sentence. The evaluation of the quality of each letter produced is based on four variables presented by the MHA (Reisman, 1999), adapted to our context. The variables assessed are legibility, shape, size, alignment of letters and spacing between letters and words. The following is a description of the criteria adopted for assessing the quality of each letter in each of the variables according to Reisman (1999), adapted to our context (Calvo et al. 2014, Pasculli, 2014).

Legibility refers to the ability to identify and interpret the symbol (letter) produced by a combination of handwriting strokes. An unreadable letter received a point of error in all five qualitative categories.

Form: refers to the characteristics of the traces of the symbol (letter), such as proportionality and sharpness of the traces.

Size: refers to the production of the letters accompanying or not all reference lines, except for the baseline. Respecting the lines above or below the base line in the manner that the size of the letters is preserved. Thus, each letter was evaluated taking into account the vertical dimensions. The height of the letters in relation to the lines was considered.

Alignment: it refers to the traces of the letters accompanying the base line, and the letters floating on the base line characterize errors of alignment.

Spacing refers to the space between letters and words. To measure the spaces between the letters and words of the sentence must be consistent and according to specific space patterns.

According to Reisman (1999), each letter can receive only one point of error in each category, even if several violations of established criteria occur. As per the author's instructions, a participant's evaluation starts with a score of 42 points maximum. Each point is deducted one point from this initial score. Thus, the higher the score achieved, the better the quality of the stroke of the letter for handwriting.

A study conducted by the authors of this chapter sought to validate and adapt cross-culturally to the Brazilian context the MHA (Pasculli, 2014). In the study by Pasculli (2014) 448 children enrolled in the 2nd and 3rd years of the public school system and two school teachers who were examiners to carry out the validation of MHA adapted to the Brazilian context participated. The results of the validation of the MHA demonstrated the satisfactory results for validation of the instrument of assessment of the handwriting stroke. Thus, the results allow stating, in general, that the Brazilian version of this instrument meets the criteria for use in the Brazilian Educational System.

CONCLUSION

The Minnesota Handwriting Assessment (Reisman, 1999) is an easy-to-administer handwriting assessment tool that can be incorporated into the procedures to be used by teachers in the process of acquisition of the handwriting skill. This type of assessment allows us to objectively assess how the quality of each child's handwriting is individual, as well as to assess the progress of each child and the class as a whole. In addition, it is possible to extract from these results which variables of the quality of the handwriting trajectory that evolved at a smaller scale and that could be the focus of attention on the part of the teachers to facilitate the process of literacy of the students.

References

Bara, F. & Gentaz, E. (2010) Haptics in teaching handwriting: The role of perceptual and visuo-motor skills. *Human Movement Science*, 30 (4), 745-759.

BRAZIL, Ministry of Education. *National Pact for Literacy in the Right Age,* 2013.

Brito, A. E. (2007) Literacy pedagogical practice: the acquisition of written language as sociocultural process. *Revista Iberoamericana de Educación,* 4 (44), 1-9.

Bumin, G. & Kavak, S. T. (2008) An investigation of the factors affecting handwriting performance in children with hemiplegic cerebral palsy. *Disability and Rehabilitation*, 30 (18), 1374-1385.

Calvo, A. P., Pasculli, A. G., Hiraga, C. Y., Del Masso, M. C., & Pellegrini, A. M. (2014) Writing quality: Intervention based on the variation of finger force production. *Cadernos de Terapia Ocupacional*, 22 (2), 317-325.

Elliot, J. M. & Connolly, K. J. (1984) A classification of manipulative hand movements. *Developmental Medicine and Child Neurology*, 26, 283-296.

Fávero, M. T. M. (2005) *Psychomotor development and learning of writing.* Dissertation (Masters in learning and teacher action). State University of Maringá, Maringá.

Feder, K. P. & Majnemer, A. (2007) Handwriting development, competency, and intervention. *Developmental Medicine & Child Neurology,* 49, 312-317.

Ferreiro, E. (1986) Literacy in process. *Creative Commons License.*

Fuentes, C. T., Mostofsky, S. H., & Bastian, A. J. (2009) Children with autism show specific handwriting impairments. *Neurology,* 73 (19), 1532-1537.

Latash, M. L., Danion, F., Scholz, J. F., Zatsiortsky, V. M., & Schöner, G. (2003) Approaches to analysis of handwriting as a coordination task to a redundant motor system. *Human Movement Science*, 22, 153-171.

Le Roux, Y. (2005) *Apprentissage de L'écriture et psychomotricité* [*Learning Writing and psychomotility*]. Marseille: Solal.

Pasculli, A. G. (2014) *Transcultural Translation and Adaptation of the Minnesota Handwriting Assessment for Application in Brazil.* Dissertation (Master of Human Development and Technologies). Institute of Biosciences, State University Paulista, Rio Claro.

Pellegrini, A. M. & Hiraga, C. Y. (2008) Intervention in the context of motor behavior: integrating theory and practice. In: Corrêa, U. C., (Org.). *Research on motor behavior: the professional intervention in perspective*. (Pp. 116-129) São Paulo: EFP/EEFEUSP.

Racine, M. B., Majnemer, A., Shevell, M., & Snider, L. (2008) Handwriting performance in children with attention deficit hyperactivity disorder (ADHD). *Journal of Child Neurology*, 23 (4), 399-406.

Reisman, J. (1999) *Minnesota Handwriting Assessment manual.* San Antonio, TX: Harcourt Assessment Inc.

Rosenblum, S., Weiss, P. L., & Parush, S. (2003) Computerized Temporal Handwriting Characteristics of Proficient and Non-proficient Hand-Writers. *The American Journal of Occupational Therapy*, 57 (2), 129-138.

Schneck, C. M. & Henderson, A. (1990) Descriptive analysis of the developmental progression for pencil and crayon control in nondysfunctional children. *The American Journal of Occupational Therapy*, 44, 893-900.

Sodrê, L. G. P. (2000) Motor development of the dominant hand in the movements identified as responsible for written production. *School Psychology and Education*, 4 (2), 21-29.

Tam, C., Ryan, S. E., Rigby, P., & Sophianopoulos, M. (2009) Rater reliability of the adapted scoring criteria of the Minnesota Handwriting Assessment for children with cerebral palsy. *Australian Occupational Therapy Journal*, 56, 403-408.

Tseng, M. H. & Cermark, S. A. (1993) The influences of ergonomic factors and perceptual motor abilities on handwriting performance. *The American Journal of Occupational Therapy*, 47, 919-926.

In: Handwriting and Dysgrafia
Editors: M. Herrera Cardoso et al.
ISBN: 978-1-53613-805-4

Chapter 4

UNDERSTANDING, DIAGNOSIS AND INTERVENTION IN DYSGRAPHIA

Marielza Regina Ismael Martins *
and José Alexandre Bastos
Boots Cat Project – São José do Rio Preto Medical School (FAMERP),
São José do Rio Preto Educational Department,
São José do Rio Preto, São Paulo, Brazil

ABSTRACT

The disorder of writing expression below the level expected for chronological age, intelligence, and schooling in specialized literature is called dysgraphia. Handwriting skills activate the brain, stimulating the reading circuit. Dysgraphia interferes with the individual's ability to express ideas, and expressive writing requires that many mental functions synchronize at the same time: organization, memory, attention, motor skills, and various aspects of linguistic skill. In this chapter we will observe that several brain systems interact to produce dysgraphia. Some experts believe that dysgraphia involves a dysfunction in the interaction between the two main brain systems that allows a person to translate

* Corresponding Author Email: marielzamartins@famerp.br

mental into written language (phonemes to graphemes translation, i.e., sound to symbol and lexicon to grapheme translation). Other studies have shown that split attention, memory load, and familiarity of graphic material affect writing ability. Typically, a person with illegible handwriting has a combination of fine motor difficulty, inability to revisualize letters, and inability to remember the motor patterns of letter forms. The assessment and intervention, also addressed in this chapter, aims at that health and education professionals should be able to identify and refer children at risk with handwriting difficulties, directing the family to seek an etiological diagnosis for timely and appropriate strategies are implemented early.

Keywords: learning disorder, dysgraphia, handwriting, evaluation, early intervention

INTRODUCTION

Since handwriting is one of the man's greatest inventions, it is considered the divisor line between pre-history and history. Man´s necessity to perennially register his daily life, his rituals and even his thoughts, has begun with the pictography. Later a figure could have several meanings: the sun would represent the light, the day and the heat, this is the so-called ideography. Handwriting was developed by the Babylonians (500 A.C.), with curve-shaped symbols drawn on the clay; the cuneiform denomination (IPHAN, 2014).

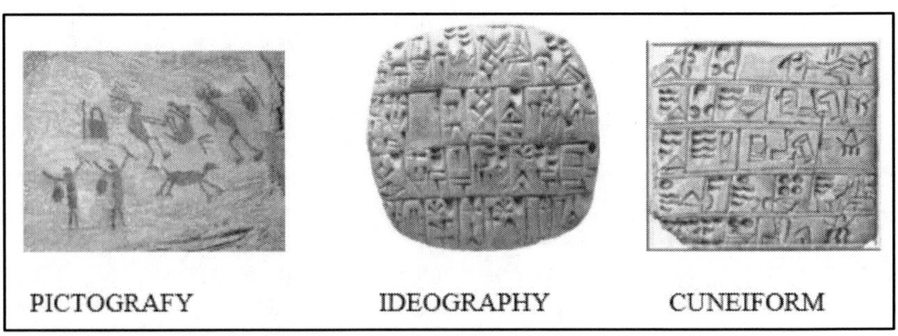

Figure 1. First types of writing.

In the course of history several peoples simultaneously developed several forms of handwrinting and reading, Portuguese language from the Latin alphabet (Metzloff, Kuhl, Movellan, & Sejnowski, 2009). Speech is acquired spontaneously by the human being, as long as his hearing is preserved and there is adequate exposure to a particular language. However, a formal way must be used to learn reading and writing; and this comprises different cerebral structures, and their development has to be progressive and the outcome will depend on multifactor (Mody, 2003).

EVOLUTION OF THE HANDWRITING

Handwriting is a complex task demanding visual-motor coordination, visual perception and kinesthetic skills (Feder & Majnemer, 2007). To learn writing involves cognition, moreover the motor learning process (Berninger, Nielsen, Abbott, Wijsman, & Raskind, 2008). Around the second year of life the child learns to keep one's pencil and scribbles up, down and in circles, the scribble is for writing what babbling is for speech. This process evolves over time: risks are vertical at the age of two, horizontal at two and a half, circle at three years. To copy a cross is at the age of four, the square at five years and the triangle at five years and a half; this can point out readiness for writing (Beery, 2010).

Since motor skill has been improving, the child uses block letters to write at first. Later cursive handwriting is used being shorter with little variation; finally, automation is acquired between eight and nine years. Difficulties with graphing skills may result in illegible handwriting compromising the child's academic performance (Feder & Majnemer, 2007). As a result the child will not be able to produce an acceptable cultural handwriting despite adequate intellectual level. This is called dysgraphia (Ajuriaguerra, 1988). (Ajuriaguerra, 1988).

CLASSIFICATION

The dysgraphia can be classified into three types, the interesting thing is that when it differs there may be variation in prognosis and treatment (Ardila & Rosselli, 1993; Torres & Fernandes, 2001; Miceli & Capasso, 2006).

1. Dyslexic dysgraphia: spontaneous writing is illegible, especially in complex texts; the spelling is compromised, but drawing and writing under copy are less compromised. Fine motor performance tests such as normal finger tapping speed.
2. Motor dysgraphia: spontaneous copying and handwriting may be illegible, drawing and abnormal finger tapping speed.
3. Spatial dysgraphia: people have illegible handwriting both in copy and spontaneous; tapping speed with finger is normal, while drawing is impaired.

Therefore, the diagnosis is not only performed by the analysis of the handwriting; tests are more comprehensive analyzing the spontaneous writing and texts according to the age.

Posture should be included during the writing routine, pencil grasp, handwriting fatigue, hand tremors in handwriting, finger speed test and pulse rotation (Feifer & Defina, 2002).

SIGNALS AND SYMPTONS

The handwriting in block and cursive letters are illegible, regardless appropriate time; block and cursive letters mixed , upward or downward irregularities and irregular letter size, incomplete words and omission of words in a sentence; gaps between words and letters. Some wrist strange movements, position of the body in front of the sheet of paper; writing on the copy is slow and laborious; poor spatial orientation on paper; pencil footprint is very strong resulting rapid fatigue; great difficulty in thinking and writing at the same time (Wolf, 2011).

The following scheme shows how motor difficulties can arise for various reasons and how information is processed and used (Missiuna et al., 2012).

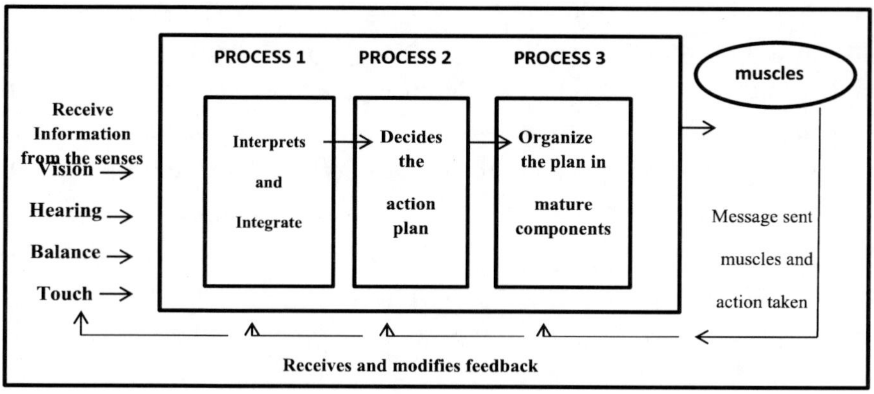

Figure 2. Activity planning system.

The child may find it difficult to analyze the sensory information from the environment; use this information to select the desired action plan; to follow up the movement task engines; send correct message to produce a coordinated action; interact all of these actions in order to control the movement while it is occurring. The result of any of these problems is the same; the child will appear troubled, clumsy, and will have difficulty learning to perform new motor tasks (Schwellnus et al., 2012).

Neuropsychology and Dysgraphia

The construct of written language involves a number of cognitive functions such as attention, spatial orientation, sequencing, memory, language, and higher cognitive command. The dysfunction of these skills leads to poor planning, erratic readability, irregular memory flow, poor self-monitoring and careless mistakes; the lack of spatial orientation leads to poor spatial orientation of the page, unequal space between letters and words, problems in organization and poor use of lines (Ruthmary & Deuel, 1995).

The sequencing disorder leads to the slow learning of motor movements in relation to block and cursive letters, poor sequence in the narrative and problem organization. Changes in memory lead to failures in word recall, fluctuation on the memory of letter motor engrams, poor handwriting, poor readability, preference for block letter rather than the cursive, and deterioration of writing skills in continuous form when compared to simple words and sentences (Zoccolotti & Friedmann, 2010).

The outcome of language changes can cause poor written expression, inadequate use of colloquial language, impoverished vocabulary and grammar confusion. Disordes in the higher cognitive command provide simplistic ideation, low development of opinion and lack of idea development (Coltheart, Rastle, Perry, Langdon, & Ziegler, 2001).

NEUROANATOMIC CORRELATION AND HANDWRITTING

As already mentioned the writing process is complex and involves several cerebral areas. It is important to reflect that the brain has not changed according to the macro and microscopic point of view in the last millennia, but had to adapt to new functions as long as inventions were developed. Writing is one of these, as the neurons of the occipito-temporal region (fusiform gyrus) had to recycle to identify letters and numbers and to transmit them to other cerebral areas, thus these symbols have meaning.

The cerebral areas and their function in the process of written language are described below: (Feifer & Defina, 2002):

- Ascending reticular system - is responsible for the level of alertness and orientation;

- Wernicke Area - is responsible for the auditory association in the temporal lobe to understand the linguistic direction in the written task;
- Temporal lobe - determines the direction of silent reading in written language tasks;
- Limbic system - gives emotional connectivity to the subject;
- Anterior cingulo circuit - focuses our inner attention;
- Hippocampus - retrieves the memories stored in the cortex in the sense of time and space;
- Medium temporal lobe - records our lexicon of words stored in the semantic code;
- Inferior parietal lobe - is the network of higher level thinking and tertiary area problem solving;
- Frontal lobe - responsible for the syntactic arrangement of thoughts and ideas in linguistic form;
- Pre-frontal dorsolateral cortex - organizes and executes thought planning, working memory to retain ideas in the mind and support of attention to manual tasks, inhibits distracting thoughts, initiates tasks and maintains motivational persistence;
- Pre-motor cortex - plans sequential motor response;
- Motor cortex - performs writing motor act; prefrontal cortex lateral dorsum - gives the self-monitoring response;
- Cerebellum - monitors the proprioceptive feedback of the motor response.

EVALUATIONS AND INTERVENTION

Brazilian studies on dysgraphia are scarce. In 2013 a descriptive, exploratory cross-sectional study was carried out on schoolchildren from the public network of the municipality of São José do Rio Preto, SP. Sixty-three (6th grade) children from 13 public schools were evaluated through the production of a thematic essay. This aimed at observing their textual production by analyzing specific characteristics, according to the Analytical Discrete Inventory (adapted) (Alvarado Gordillo, 1988). This is used to recognize the difficulties of handwriting through the graphic drawing (unrecognizable letters; graphics that allow the confusion of letters, angulations, retouched letters, abnormal patterns of letters, ascending/descending and floating line). Children with vision and hearing impaired, chronic diseases and subnormal intelligence were excluded. In this study, one hundred and thirty-eight children have presented all signs of dysgraphia. If the indicators were correlated to gender, the boys were the prevalent and the predominant co-occurrence was dyslexia (Martins et al., 2013).

International literature on dysgraphia is comprehensive, while it is reduced in Brazil. These studies have been investigating dysgraphia by observing writing speed (production rate). Legibility of the letter in relation to shape, alignment, spacing and dimension, as well as observing fatigue in writing, socioeconomic level among others (Summers & Catarro, 2003). It is also oberved associations with other disorders such as autism spectrum disorder (Fuentes, Mostofsky, & Bastian, 2009); developmental coordination disorder (Santos & Vieira, 2013) and attention deficit hyperactivity disorder (Frings et al. 2010).

The tests, inventories, protocols are inserted in three commonly used methods which are global-holistic assessments, which are based on whether a product is written and readable or illegible comparing with a group of standard samples (Rosenblum, Chevion, & Weiss, 2006 Li-Tsang et al., 2011); analytical assessments that presuppose a relationship between performance criteria (format and space of letters and words, alignment, scaling) and readability, assessing each criterion individually and calculating a global score (Rosenblum, Parush, & Weiss 2003; Li-Tsang et al., 2011), and computerized measurements (Rosenblum, Weiss, & Parush, 2004).

The computerized methods that use the technology for writing comprehension are also widely used, and among them the Perceived Efficacy and Goal Setting System (PEGS) (Missiuna, Pollock, Law, Walter, & Cavey, 2006), the Computerized Permanship Evaluation Tool

(ComPet) (Rosenblum, Weiss & Parush, 2004) and the Chinese Handwriting Assessment Tool (CHAT) (Li-Tsang et al., 2011), which is widely used in scientific research.

In Brazil, specific assessment tools based on adequate criteria for school-age children are insufficient. The most used are the Scale of Dysgraphia (Lorenzini, 1993) that adapted it from the Ajuriaguerra Scale Scale, the Analytical Discrete Inventory (Alvarado Gordillo, 1998) and the McMaster Protocol of Writing Evaluation (Pollock et al., 2009). All these for research purposes only. The Detailed Assessment of writing speed - DASH (Cardoso, 2014) is being validated.

INTERVENTION

After evaluation and identification of the type of dysgraphia as a function of symptoms, one should intervene by approaching the praxis dimension with improved spelling (motor dysgraphia's) and linguistic dimension intervening in the coding (dyslexic dysgraphia) and construction of meaning (written expression problems).

External factors may influence the lack of writing functionality. Thus, basic elements should be considered and evaluated such as: postural control (90-90-90 posture with feet flat on the floor, forearms supported and elbows slightly projected off the edge of the wallet and 5cm above the elbows flexed when the child is seated); support (appropriate height of the table; central sheet for right-handers slightly shifted to the right with respect to the trunk axis and inclined to the left at an angle above 45°: sheet slightly tilted to left for left-handers with angle less than 45°); tools (position the pencil tilted between 45 and 60 degrees for the table and leaning on the hand of the arch formed between the thumb and the index finger, at the beginning of preference to the three-sided pencil, larger individuals use fine-tipped pens); movements (promote the dynamic tripod hold, increase awareness about the pressure exerted on the paper, promote dissociation between finger, forearm-forearm and trunk, proper paper tilt, effective stabilization of paper with non-dominant hand) (Rigal, 2006).

Regarding behavior aspects such as endurance, attention and motivation can significantly affect writing performance. Fatigue has an effect on writing speed, letter form, organization and ergonomics (Coallier & Rouleau, 2014).

Thus evaluating and intervening in writing must attend semantic processes - ability to plan writing; syntactic processes - ability to construct prayers; Lexical processes - centralized in the recovery and access to words in both reading and writing, and in motor processes - related to the reading process (Rosenblum, Weiss, Parush, 2004).

Three fundamental factors should be considered for the reeducation of graphics: *psychomotor development* with the aim to train aspects related to posture, body control, movement dissociation, mental representation of gesture required for the trait, spatial-temporal perception, lateralization and visual-motor coordination. The *development of graphics* by itself; the professional must differentiate pictographic activities (painting, drawing, modeling) and writing (the use of pencil and paper to improve movements and graphic position) and should correct errors characteristic of the graphics, such as shape, size and slope of the letters, the aspect of the text, the inclination of the paper and the maintenance of the margins and lines (Coelho, 2013). Finally, the *specificity of graphics* aims at correcting specific errors in the graphics of that descriptive child: it includes letterforms, letter size, letter slope, links, text aspect, paper slope, margin maintenance, among other factors (Karlsdottir & Stefansson, 2002).

No consensus about the preferred letter for handwriting is observed in the literature, but Adelantado (2004) pointed out the cursive handwriting to dysgraphic children, since the script letter presents some difficulty in detecting word separation, slowness and ease of inversions. Psychomotor intervention in dysgraphia is the most commonly used approach, since finger-manual reeducation aims to achieve precision in the hand domain, avoiding involuntary movements in certain muscle groups. This can improve dissociation and flexibility of digital movements as well as the coordination and adaptation of manual movements on writing, thus improving the graphical execution (Torres & Fernandes, 2001).

Some basic manual exercises account for the awareness of the gestures such as the movement of closing and opening wrists, union and separation of the hands, movements of gesture imitation, throwing and catching balls and alternating the hands on different tasks, one hand hitting the head and another rubbing the stomach. Also exercises that provide independence of the fingers (closing the hand and stretching the fingers one by one, tapping the fingers); and digital coordination on fine motor skills - strings to knot, to do and undo knots, among others (Berninger & Wolf, 2009).

Since the oculomotor coordination is necessary for a good graphic quality in writing, visual-motor coordination to improve the articulation of the hand movements with visual perception is stimulated. Some exercises can be used to favor the dissociation of manual movements, training to grasp the pencil. At the same time, they stimulate visual perception: perforated or punctured, observing the figure contour, drawings and lines; cut or tear, also made on drawings, figures and lines; threaded keys in perforated frames; attach parts to docking trays, thread perforated balls into a wire).

Finally, the reeducation of graphism that guides the development of abilities and skills related to handwriting seek to correct the spelling mistakes through grip and pressure exercises. These exercises teach the child to properly hold the pencil and which pressure to apply, which should be sufficient, but moderate, favoring fluidity of movement and uniform trace. Exercises of automation of left-right movements; exercises on straight lines and curves; exercises on mixed lines; and exercise drawings contours. These exercises have a sequence that motor activities go from the global to the finest. First, they must be performed in the air and then in tissues, using the digitate, so that the child acquires sufficient control and interiorization of the movements. After this phase you move to exercises in graphic spaces.

REFERENCES

Adelantado, P. (2004). Entendiendo la disgrafia: El ajuste visomotor em la escritura manual [Understanding dysgraphia: Visual motor adjustment in manual writing]. *Revista Iberamericana Psicomotricidad y Tecnicas Corporales*, 14(3), 39-67.

Ajuriaguerra, J et al., A escrita infantil: evolução e dificuldades [A children's written: evolution and difficulties]. Porto Alegre: Artes Médicas; 1988. 301p.

Alvarado Gordillo, M. (1988). *La disgrafía escolar: escala disgráfica, tratamientos correctivos* [*School dysgraphia: dysgraphic scale, corrective treatments*]. Alicante: Editorial Disgrafos; 109p.

Ardila, A. & Rosselli, M. (1993). Spatial agraphia. *Brain Cognition*, 22, 137-147.

Beery KE, Beery NA. *The Beery-Buktenica Developmental Test of Visual-Motor Integration. 6 ed.* Texas: Pearson; 2010. 209p.

Berninger, V. W., Nielsen, K. H., Abbott, R. D., Wijsman, E., & Raskind W. (2008). Gender differences in severity of writing and reading disabilities. *Journal School Psychology*, 46, 151-72.

Berninger, V. & Wolf, B. (2009). *Teaching students with dyslexia and dysgraphia: Lessons from teaching and science.* Baltimore, MD: Paul H. Brookes.

Biblioteca Aloisio Magalhaes – *IPHAN (2014) - A história da escrita* [*IPHAN (2014) - A story written*]. https://biblioam.wordpress.com/ 2014/08/22/a-historia-da-escrita/.

Cardoso, M. H. (2014). *Adaptação cultural do Detailed Assessment of Speed of Handwriting (DASH) para escolares de ensino público* [*Cultural Adaptation of Detailed Assessment of Speed of Handwriting (DASH) for schoolchildren in the public sphere*]. Dissertação - Universidade Estadual Paulista, Faculdade de Filosofia e Ciências, Marilia.

Coallier, M. & Rouleau, N. (2014).Visual-Motor Skills Performance on the Beery VMI: A Study of Canadian Kindergarten Children. *The Open Journal of Occupational Therapy*, 2(2), Article 4.

Coelho, D. (2013) *Dificuldades de Aprendizagem específicas: Dislexia, Disgrafia, Disortografia e Discalculia* [*Specific Apprentice Dificities: Dyslexia, Dysgraphia, Disortography and Dyscalculia*]. Porto: Areal Editoras. 224p.

Coltheart, M., Rastle, K., Perry, C., Langdon, R., & Ziegler, T. (2001) DRC: Dual-route cascaded model of visual word recognition and reading aloud. *Psychological Review*, 108, 204-256.

Erez, N., Yochman, A., & Parush, S. (1999) *The Hebrew Handwriting Evaluation* (2nd ed.). Israel: School of Occupational Therapy, Faculty of Medicine, Hebrew University of Jerusalem.

Feder, K. P. & Majnemer, A. (2007). Handwriting development, Competency and intervention. *Developmental Medicine Child Neurology*; 49: 312-7.

Feifer, S. G & Defina, P. D. (2002). *The neuropsychology of written language disorders: diagnosis and intervention.* Middletown MD: School .Neuropsych Press.

Frings, M., Gaertner, K., Buderath, P., Christiansen, H., Gerwig, M., Hein-Kropp, C. et al. (2010). Megalographia in children with cerebellar lesions and in children with attention deficit/hyperactivity disorder. *The Cerebellum*, 9, 429–432.

Fuentes, C., Mostofsky, S., & Bastian, A. (2009) Children with autism show specific handwriting impairments. *Neurology,* 73(4), 1532–1537.

Karlsdottir, R. & Stefansson, T. (2002). Problems in developing functional handwriting. *Perceptual Motor Skills*, 94(2), 623-62.

Li-Tsang, C., Au, R. K., Chan, M. H., Chan, L. W., Lau, G. M., Lo, T. K. et al., (2011) Handwriting characteristics among secondary students with and without physical disabilities: A study with a computerized tool. *Research in Developmental Disabilities,* 32 (1), 207–216.

Lorenzini M. (1993). *Uma escala para detectar a disgrafia baseada na escala de Ajuriaguerra* [*A scale to detect dysgraphia based on the Ajuriaguerra scale*]. Dissertação– Programa de Pós-Graduação em Fisioterapia, Universidade Federal de São Carlos, São Carlos.

Martins, M., Bastos, J., Cecato, A., Araujo, M., Magro, R., & Alaminos, V. (2013). Rastreio de disgrafia motora em escolares da rede pública de ensino [Role of motor dysgraphia in schools of the public network of Ensino]. *Journal de Pediatria*, 89(1), 70-74.

Metzloff, A. N., Kuhl, P. K., Movellan, J., & Sejnowski, T. J. (2009). Foundations for a New Science of Learning. *Science*, 325, 284-288.

Miceli, G. & Capasso, R. (2006). Spelling and dysgrafia. *Cognitive Neuropsycology*, 23(1), 110-134.

Missiuna, C. A., Pollock, N. A., Levac, D. E., Campbell, W. N., Whalen, S. D., Bennett, S. M. et al., (2012). Partnering for change: an innovative school-based occupational therapy service delivery model for children with developmental coordination disorder. *Canadian Journal Occupational Therapy*, 79(1), 41-50.

Missiuna, C., Pollock, N., Law, M., Walter, S., & Cavey, N. (2006). Examination of the Perceived Efficacy and Goal Setting System (PEGS) with children with disabilities, their parents, and teachers. *American Journal of Occupational Therapy,* 60, 204–214.

Mody, M. (2003) Phonological basis in reading disabilitiy: A review and analysis of the evidence. *Reading and writing: an interdisciplinary Journal*. 16:21-9.

Pollock, N., Lockhart, J., Blowes, B., Semple, K., Webster, M., Farhat, L. et al., (2009). *Protocolo McMaster de Avaliação da Escrita (2 ed.)* [*McMaster Protocol of Avaliação da Escrita (2 ed.)*]. Trad. L.C. Magalhães, A. P. F. Costa, S. A. Capellini, & P. M. M Okuda. Universidade McMaster. Disponível em: <https://public.canchild.ca/inventory/readmore/5194bc86-bac2-4fd6-94d7-520f4330a2e4> Acesso em: 02 abril 2016.

Reisman, J. (1999). *Minnesota Handwriting Assessment*. San Antonio, TX: The Psychological Corporation.

Rigal, R. (2006). *Educacion motriz y educacion psicomotriz en pré-escolar y primaria (1 ed.)* [*Motor education and psychomotor education in pre-school and primary (1 ed.)*]. Espanha: INDE Publicaciones.

Rosenblum, S., Parush, S., & Weiss, P. (2003). Computerized temporal handwriting characteristics of proficient and non-proficient handwriters. *The American Journal of Occupational Therapy*, 57(2), 129–138.

Rosenblum, S. (2008) Development, reliability, and validity of the Handwriting Proficiency Screening Questionnaire (HPSQ). *American Journal of Occupational Therapy,* 62, 298–307.

Rosenblum, S., Chevion, D., & Weiss, P. L. (2006). Using data visualization and signal processing to characterize the handwriting process. *Pediatric Rehabilitation*, 9(4):404-17.

Rosenblum, S., Weiss, P., & Parush, S. (2004). Handwriting evaluation for developmental dysgrafia: Process versus. Product. *Interdisciplinary Journal*, 17(5), 433- 458.

Ruthmary K. & Deuel, M. D. (1995). Developmental Dysgraphia and Motor Skills Disorders. *Journal of child Neurology*, 10 (1), S6-S8.

Santos, P. & Vieira, L. (2013). Prevalência de desordem coordenativa desenvolvimental em crianças com 7 a 10 anos de idade. *Revista Brazileira de Cineantropometria e Desempenho Humano* [Prevalence of desordem coordenativa desenvolvimental em crianças com 7 to 10 years of idade. *Brazilian Magazine of Cineanthropology and Human Dignity*], 15(2), 233–242.

Schwellnus, H., Carnahan, H., Kushki, A., Polatajko, H., Missiuna, C., & Chau, T. (2012). Effect of pencil grasp on the speed and legibility of handwriting after a 10-minute copy task in Grade 4 children. *Australian Occupational Therapy Journal,* 59(3), 180-7.

Summers, J. & Catarro, F. (2003). Assessment of handwriting speed and factors influencing written output of university students in examinations. *Australian Occupational Therapy Journal*, 50(3), 148-157.

Torres, R. M. & Fernandez, P. F. (2001). *Dislexia, disortografia e disgrafia* [*Dyslexia, disortography and dysgraphia*]. Lisboa: McGraw-Hill; p. 188.

Wolf, B. (2011). Teaching handwriting. In J. Birsch (Ed.), *Multisensory teaching of basic language skills: Theory and practice*, Revised Edition. Baltimore, MD: Paul H. Brookes.

Zoccolotti, P. & Friedmann, N. (2010). From dyslexia to dyslexias, from dysgraphia to dysgraphias, from a cause to causes: A look at current research on developmental dyslexia and dysgraphia. *Cortex*, 46(10), 1211-1215.

In: Handwriting and Dysgrafia
Editors: M. Herrera Cardoso et al. ISBN: 978-1-53613-805-4

Chapter 5

APPLICATION OF THE DETAILED ASSESSMENT OF SPEED OF HANDWRITING (DASH) TO BRAZILIAN STUDENTS

Monique Herrera Cardoso[1,*] and Simone Aparecida Capellini[2,†]

[1] Education Program,
São Paulo State University "Júlio de Mesquita Filho" (UNESP),
Marília, São Paulo, Brazil

[2] Department of Speech and Hearing Sciences,
São Paulo State University "Júlio de Mesquita Filho" (UNESP),
Marília, São Paulo, Brazil

ABSTRACT

This chapter aims to present the speed of writing, according to readability, of Brazilian public school students. Thus, the Brazilian Adaptation of the Detailed Assessment of Speed of Handwriting was

* Graduate Student; Corresponding Author: moniquehc@gmail.com
† Full-Professor

applied to 658 students of both genders, aged from 09 to 16 years and 11 months, of 05 public schools. The legible words were identified by means of analyzes carried out by expert judges in handwriting, and the illegible ones were excluded. The speed calculation took into account only the legible words, divided by the time of each proposed task. It can be observed that: in general, the writing speed increases according to the increase of the age group; 12-year-old students present lower writing speed during copy activities when compared to younger students; students aged from 14 to 15 years, present lower writing speed during free-writing and quick-graph activities when compared to younger students; the cognitive and linguistic requirements in each task of the procedure are different, which resulted in the decrease of the writing speed, according to each task. The present findings contemplate the expected results, in terms of written proficiency for each age group, however, new studies on the reliability and validity of the instrument for the Brazilian population are necessary.

Keywords: manual writing, speech therapy, assessment

INTRODUCTION

Even in modern times, in which technology is advancing more and more, it can observed that mastering writing skills still constitutes an important goal that students must achieve (Mccarney, Peters, Jackson, Thomas, Kirby, 2013), and therefore requires more attention from educators and health professionals (Feder & Majnemer, 2007), as it plays a crucial role in school performance, with important implications for the motor and cognitive development (Accardo, Genna, & Borean, 2013).

According to the study by Overvelde and Hulstijn (2011) writing becomes automatic and organized around 8-9 years, being establishing as an available tool to facilitate the development of ideas of the students. However, it is common to observe students who were submitted to writing practice in primary education, presenting difficulties in producing a comprehensive writing, whose readability (quality), and speed (production rate) are impaired. Francis, Wallen, & Bundy (2016) state in their study that writing speed constitutes an important component of students' ability to properly express their ideas, knowledge and creativity in an effective way.

However, from 10 to 30% of the students present difficulties in following the development of writing (Feder & Majnemer, 2007) and, therefore, tend to be frustrated in trying to put their ideas on the paper, inhibiting their ability to compose texts (Medwell & Wray, 2008). Continuous difficulties can lead to low self-esteem and less motivation for trying to improve your writing, especially when workload increases as schooling progresses (Martins et al., 2013).

When the student is competent in other areas, issues of difficulty concerning writing can be attributed to laziness or lack of motivation, rather than a specific learning difficulty, which affects the production of the language in its written form (Berninger, Abbott, Augsburger, & Garcia, 2009).

In Brazil, it is difficult to identify the students who actually present difficulties regarding the quality of manual writing, because the calligraphy teaching methodology is not standardized, so, each school emphasizes and defines its practice, and also, due to the lack of specific evaluation tools based on adequate criteria for Brazilian school-age students, to measure the speed of performance and to observe the writing readability aspects.

The Detailed Assessment of Speed of Handwriting - DASH (Barnett, Henderson, Scheib, & Schulz, 2007) is an example of an instrument which proposes to evaluate the speed of writing, taking into account the readability. It is a standardized procedure with a representative stratified sample from the UK, and identifies students aged from 9 to 16 years with writing difficulties due to inadequate speed, providing a reliable measure of age-appropriate writing speed and a detailed description of the writing performance. It is also applied to control the intervention programs' therapeutic efficacy.

It is composed of five tasks : four writing tasks (Task 1 – Copy best, Task 2 – Alphabet writing, Task 3 – Copy fast, Task 5 - Free thematic writing), and one of them consists on the measure of perceptual- motor competence, that is, it does not involve the language linguistic aspects (Task 4 – Graphic speed).

The cross-cultural adaptation of DASH (Barnett et al., 2007) to the Brazilian population can be checked in the study by Cardoso, Herderson and Capellini (2014), which concluded that this procedure could be applied to the population. Therefore, this chapter aims to investigate the speed of writing, according to the readability of the Brazilian public school students.

It is believed that the use of instruments based on normality criteria can help health and education professionals to evaluate the quality of writing, to diagnose delay in writing development as well as dysgraphia.

MATERIAL AND METHOD

This study was submitted to the Research Ethics Committee of the Faculty of Philosophy and Sciences of the São Paulo State University - CEP/FFC/UNESP/Marília - SP and was approved, according to protocol number 0444/2012.

This study was carried out in 5 public schools, located in the city of Marília (SP) and in the Region; one state school, and one was municipal in a region considered as rural, one state school and one municipal in the south region; and one municipal in the north region. These schools took part of training sessions carried out by the Investigation Learning Disabilities Laboratory (LIDA) of the Department of Speech and Hearing Therapy at Unesp, in Marília (SP). Consequently, their schoolchildren are often accompanied by the whole team (pedagogues, speech therapists, occupational therapists, neuropsychologists, neuropediatricians and psychopedagogues) and, therefore, diagnosed and referred to intervention, when necessary.

The students selected to participate in this study should be aged between 9 years and 16 years and 11 months, deliver the Free and Informed Consent signed by the parents or guardians, and should not have notes referring to presence of sensory, motor or cognitive and/or constant auditory, visual or motor complaint in their school records. Failure to comply with at least one of the criteria described above automatically excluded the student from the study sample.

As selection criteria, a cognitive evaluation test (Raven - Raven, Raven, & Court, 1988) was applied to exclude cases of mental retardation, as well as a survey was carried out with the pedagogical coordinators about the students who presented school complaints (e.g., autism, ADHD, dyslexia, among others), being excluded from the data sample of this study.

According to the criteria, 658 students of both genders participated in the age group from 09 years to 16 years and 11 months of age, being divided into age groups (Table 1).

Data collection of the students was performed in groups of 15 to 20 students in a single session, not exceeding 50 minutes. Students should use standard lined sheets, their own pencils and rubber.

To calculate the writing speed of the students, considering writing readability, it was initially necessary, to identify the legible words (step 1). After the identification it was possible to calculate the writing speed (step 2), which is the purpose of this study.

Table 1. Distribution of the number of students evaluated according to the study groups, age group and gender

Groups	Age	N	Male		Female	
			N	(%)	N	(%)
GI	09 years to 09 years and 11 months	102	58	57	44	43
GII	10 years to 10 years and 11 months	99	44	44	55	56
GIII	11 years to 11 years and 11 months	86	41	47	45	53
GIV	12 years to 12 years and 11 months	90	43	48	47	52
GV	13 years to 13 years and 11 months	87	39	45	48	55
GVI	14 years to 14 years and 11 months	68	28	41	40	59
GVII	15 years to 15 years and 11 months	61	27	44	34	56
GVIII	16 years to 16 years and 11 months	65	34	52	31	48
Total		658	314	47.65	344	52.35

Step 1 – Definition of Legible Words

In order to obtain reliable results, the writing samples of the students were judged according to readability by four professionals who work with calligraphy and analysis of the spelling of students: a speech therapist, two occupational therapists and a pedagogue, that is, professionals who share the same concepts about calligraphy, but they act in different areas. Four judges were selected for precaution, in case any of them could not carry out the analysis within the time proposed by the researcher.

The judges should carry out the reading of each word written by the student, only once. If they did not understand, they should not insist on re-reading, or "trying" to understand using the context of the sentence. Each word in which the judge easily decoded, regardless of the context of the sentence, it was classified as legible. Sometimes, there would be misleading letters within a word, which, if considered out of the word, they would not be legible. However, if the whole word were still legible, it should be classified as such.

The Cronbach Alfa Statistical Test (or, simplified, *Cronbach's Test*) was applied to verify the level of reliability in terms of the so-called 'internal consistency' of the observed values. This, in turn, presented a variation from 0,700 to 1,000 for all variables analyzed by the judges, considering a sample with 'high' reliability levels, interpreting this task as a non-biased sample.

After this step, it can be inferred that the concept of legibility is not divergent among professionals and, therefore, the analysis of the pedagogic judge was selected to be applied in the calculation of speed (step 2).

Step 2 – Calculate Writing Speed

The calculation of writing speed was performed according to the performance that each group studied presented in each proposed task, taking into account the legibility, that is, the number of words considered legible. To know:

- In tasks 01 and 03 (Copy best and Copy fast, respectively), the speed was calculated by the total sum of words divided by two (due to two minutes of test), thus obtaining the speed of words per minute (wpm, for each of the two tasks.
- In task 02 (alphabet writing) the speed was calculated by the amount of letters the student wrote within one minute. Non-lowercase, non-cursive letters, and the letters which were not in alphabetic order were excluded (as proposed in the original procedure).
- In task 04 (Graphic speed) the speed was calculated by the sum of "x," which the student realized inside the circles. For calculation speed in this task, the "x" performed incorrectly were excluded.
- In task 05 (Free thematic writing) the speed was calculated by the total sum of legible words written during the task, divided by 10 minutes (total time of the test).

RESULTS

The speed found for each age group of Brazilian students when applying DASH tasks are described below.

It can be observed that in general, the speed of writing increases as the students get older. But in the copy tasks (copy best and copy fast), 12-year-old students showed a small decline. This fact was also evidenced for students aged 14 and 15 years in free thematic writing and graphic speed tasks.

It is also observed in Table 2, when comparing the writing speed for each task in each group, the speed was higher for Graphic Speed Task, followed by the Alphabet Writing Task, and Copy Tasks (Copy Best and Copy fast), and finally the Free Thematic Writing Task.

Table 2. Writing speed (word per minute/wpm) in each task

Group by age		Copy best	Copy fast	Alphabet writing	Free thematic writing	Graphic speed
9 years	media	10.50	13.11	17.87	7.89	28.96
	SD	3.08	3.31	5.88	2.78	11.05
10 years	media	12.99	16.21	20.35	9.30	33.30
	SD	4.63	4.35	8.62	3.47	10.26
11 years	media	14.55	18.92	21.31	9.41	34.41
	SD	4.28	4.59	10.18	2.98	13.84
12 years	media	14.11	18.61	21.40	10.51	34.83
	SD	4.36	4.40	10.52	3.93	12.49
13 years	media	15.45	20.61	21.72	11.17	38.37
	SD	4.58	3.87	10.64	3.70	17.46
14 years	media	18.10	21.64	21.81	10.62	37.15
	SD	5.15	5.06	11.52	4.12	15.26
15 years	media	18.73	22.18	22.39	9.62	33.03
	SD	4.78	4.18	10.35	4.19	13.93
16 years	media	19.11	23.43	27.83	11.12	37.95
	SD	4.90	4.96	13.30	4.19	14.14

DISCUSSION

This increase in speed as the students get older, can be justified, because at the beginning of the learning process, the movements are slow and guided by visual and kinesthetic feedbacks (Chartrel & Vinter, 2006). That is, during manual writing, information such as: the pressure exerted on the pencil and paper, the positioning of the fingers and the hand, the direction of the pencil movements and mistakes made, are stored in memory to be remembered when writing again (Almeida, Sorensen, Magna, Cruz, Ferrigno, 2013). With practice, writing becomes automatic and control of coordinated writing movements are improved with age and schooling, favoring an increase in writing speed (Sovik, 1993).

However, from ages 14 to 15, the speed tends to decrease because the concern goes beyond calligraphy, since the requirements are related to planning and revision of the written text (Kim, AlOtaiba, & Wanzek, 2015) which are the most critical for writing performance (Bourdin & Fayol, 2002), thus guaranteeing a better written text (Alves, Castro, & Olive, 2008).

However, for the decline in the writing speed of 12-year-old students when comparing with younger students during copy activities, it becomes necessary to evaluate the visual perception skills, visual closure skills, and manipulation skills with hands, because according to the literature (Brown & Link, 2016) these abilities seem to be significant writing speed predictors\for school-age student.

The results found in the comparison between the tests can be justified due to the increase of the cognitive load associated with the specific tasks. This is because the free thematic writing task, for example, requires the student the ability of writing from his memory, where the cognitive and linguistic processes (planning, semantic retrieval, spelling, etc.) are competing for limited resources of the working memory (Berninger & Amtmann, 2003).

Copy tasks (Task 01 and 03) provide a visual feedback to the writer, which in turn, reduces the spelling requirements and retrieval of letters in memory, enabling the student to "imitate" what he is seeing (Levine, 1993).

The Alphabet writing (task 02) implies in finding the form of the letter stored in memory and accessing the motor planning, establishing the parameters to execute it (Viviani, 1994), thus, requiring less cognitive processes than the other tasks written above.

Graphic speed (task 04), due to being a perceptual-motor task, does not require cognitive and linguistic processes, favoring a faster speed than the other tasks.

CONCLUSION

The main results were:

- In general, writing speed increases, according to the increase of the age group
- 12-year-old students present lower writing speed during copy activities when compared to younger students
- 14 and 15-year-old students present lower writing speed during free-writing and fast-paced activities, when compared to younger students.
- The cognitive and linguistic requirements in each task of the procedure are different; which resulted in a decrease in writing speed, according to each task.

The findings of this study contemplate the expected, in terms of writing proficiency for each age group for the five DASH tasks, however, it becomes necessary to establish new studies regarding reliability and validity of the instrument for the Brazilian population.

ACKNOWLEDGMENTS

To Pearson Assessment, a division of Pearson Education Ltd. and the Foundation for Research Support of São Paulo state (FAPESP), process number 2012/04513-0.

REFERENCES

Accardo, A. P., Genna, M., & Borean, M. (2013). Development, maturation and learning influence on handwriting kinematics. *Human*

Movement Science, 32(1), 136–146. doi: 10.1016/j.humov.2012.10.004.

Almeida, P. H. T. Q., Sorensen, C. B. S., Magna L.A., Cruz, D. M. C., & Ferrigno, I. S. V. (2013). Avaliação da escrita através da fotogrametria – estudo da preensão trípode dinâmica. *Revista de Terapia Ocupacional da Universidade de São Paulo* [Evaluation of writing through photogrammetry - study of dynamic tripod hold. *Occupational Therapy Journal of the University of São Paulo*], 24(1), 38-47. doi: http://dx.doi.org/10.11606/issn.2238-6149.v24i1p38-47.

Alves, R. A., Castro, S. L., & Olive, T. (2008). Execution and pauses in writing narratives: processing time, cognitive effort and typing skill. *International Journal of Psychology,* 43(6), 969-79. doi: 10.1080/00207590701398951.

Barnett, A. L., Henderson, S. E., Scheib, B., & Schulz, J. *Detailed Assessment of Speed of Handwriting (DASH).* United Kingdom: Person, 2007.

Berninger, V. W., Abbott, R. D., Augsburger, A., Garcia, N. (2009). Comparison of pen and keyboard transcription modes in children with and without learning disabilities. *Learning Disability Quarterly*, 32(3), 123–141. doi: 10.2307/27740364.

Berninger, V., & Amtmann, D. (2003). Preventing written expression disabilities through hearly and continuing assessment and intervention for handwriting and/or spelling problems: Research into practice. In H. Swanson, K. Harris, S. Graham (Eds.). (323-344). *Handbook of learning disabilities.* New York: Guilford Press.

Bourdin, B., & Fayol, M. (2002). Even in adults written production is still more costly than oral production. *International Journal of Psychology,* 37(4), 219-227. doi: 10.1080/00207590244000070.

Brown T., & Link, J. (2016). The association between measures of visual perception, visual-motor integration, and in-hand manipulation skills of school-age children and their manuscript handwriting speed. *British Journal of Occupational Therapy*, 79(3), 163-171. doi:10.1177/0308022615600179.

Cardoso, M. H., Henderson, S., & Capellini, S. A. (2014). Tradução e adaptação cultural Brazileira do Detailed Assessment of Speed of Handwriting: equivalência conceitual e semântica [Brazilian Translation and Adaptation of the Detailed Assessment of Speed of Handwriting: Conceptual and Semantic Equivalence]. *Audiology - Communication Research,* 19(4), 321-326. http://dx.doi.org/10.1590/S2317-64312014000400001447.

Chartrel, E., & Vinter, A. (2006). Rôle des informations visuelles dans la production de lettres cursives chez l'enfant et l'adulte. *L'année Psychologique* [Book of information about the production of cursive letters in children and adults. *The Psychological Year*], 106(1), 43–63.

Feder, K. P., & Majnemer, A. (2007). Handwriting development, competency, and intervention. *Developmental Medicine and Child Neurology*, 49(4), 312–317. http://dx.doi.org/10.1111/j.1469-8749.2007.00312.x.

Francis, A. Wallen, M., & Bundy, A. (2016). Comparison of the Properties of the Handwriting Speed Test (HST) and Detailed Assessment of Speed of Handwriting (DASH): An Exploratory Study. *Physical & Occupational Therapy in Pediatrics*. doi: 10.1080/01942638.2016.1185499.

Kim, Y. S., Al Otaiba, S., & Wanzek, J. (2015). Kindergarten predictors of third grade writing. *Learning and Individual Differences*, 37, 27–37. doi:10.1016/j.lindif.2014.11.009.

Levine, M. (1993). *Developmental Variation and Learning Disorders.* MA: Educators Pub, Cambridge.

Martins M. R., Bastos, J. A., Cecato, A. T., Araujo, M. L., Magro, R. R., Alaminos, V. (2013). Screening for motor dysgraphia in public schools. *Journal of Pediatrics* (Rio J), 89, 70-74. http://dx.doi.org/10.1016/j.jped.2013.02.011.

McCarney, D., Peters, L., Jackson, S., Thomas, M., & Kirby, A. (2013). Does Poor Handwriting Conceal Literacy Potential in Primary School Children? *International Journal of Disability, Development and Education*, 60(2), 105-118. doi:10.1080/1034912X.2013.786561.

Medwell, J., & Wray, D. (2008). Handwriting – A forgotten language skill? *Language and Education*, 22, 34–47. doi: 10.2167/le722.0.

Overvelde, A., & Hulstijn, W. (2011). Handwriting development in Grade 2 and Grade 3 primary school children with normal, at risk, or dysgraphic characteristics. *Research in Developmental Disabilities*, 32, 540–548. http://dx.doi.org/10.1016/j.ridd.2010.12.027.

Raven, J. C., Raven, J., & Court, J. H. (1988). *Matrizes Progressivas Coloridas de Raven. Manual.* São Paulo: Casa do Psicólogo.

Sovik, N. (1993). Development of children's writing performance: Some educational implications. In A. F. Kalverboer, B. Hopkins, & R. Geuze (Eds.). (229–246). *Motor development in early and later childhood: Longitudinal approaches*. New York: Cambridge University Press.

Viviani, P. (1994). Les habiletés motrices. In M. Richelle, J. Requin, & M. Robert (Eds.) (777–844), *Traité de psychologie expérimentale* [*Treaty of experimental psychology*]. Paris: PUF.

In: Handwriting and Dysgrafia
Editors: M. Herrera Cardoso et al.
ISBN: 978-1-53613-805-4

Chapter 6

THE QUALITY OF HANDWRITING OF ELEMENTARY SCHOOL STUDENTS II: A COMPARISON BETWEEN BOYS AND GIRLS

Monique Herrera Cardoso[1,*]*, *Gabriela Franco dos Santos Liporaci[2,*]* *and Simone Aparecida Capellini[3,†]

[1]Education Program,
São Paulo State University "Júlio de Mesquita Filho" (UNESP),
Marília, São Paulo, Brazil

[2]Speech Language Pathology Program,
São Paulo State University "Júlio de Mesquita Filho" (UNESP),
Marília, São Paulo, Brazil

[3]Department of Speech and Hearing Sciences,
São Paulo State University "Júlio de Mesquita Filho" (UNESP),
Marília, São Paulo, Brazil

* Graduate Student; Corresponding Author: moniquehc@gmail.com

† Full Professor; Corresponding Author: gabrielafsliporaci@gmail.com; sacap@uol.com.br

Abstract

To study and investigate the performance of the quality of handwriting of elementary school students, allows professionals, both in educational and clinical environment, the knowledge of the development of writing as well as its readability. From the context of analyzing genders, the purpose of this study was : (1) To verify if there are differences between the genders, concerning the evaluation of the quality of the written expression of primary school students II; (2) To verify if there is gender prevalence regarding the diagnosis of dysgraphia. A total of 96 students of both genders, aged 11 to 14 years and 11 months, enrolled from the sixth to the ninth grade of elementary school II of a public school, took part in this study. The students were divided according to their respective school grades. Data collection was performed on a single day, inside the room, in the presence of the teacher and the researcher, not exceeding 20 minutes of activity. As procedure, the Dysgraphia Scale was used. The results presented in this study showed that male students tend to present greater difficulties regarding calligraphy, when compared to female students of elementary school II. Although no statistically significant difference was found for dysgraphia, it was possible to identify only male students with this diagnosis.

Keywords: manual writing, dysgraphia, written language

Introduction

Mastering writing skills is still an important goal that students must achieve (McCarney, Peters, Jackson, Thomas, & Kirby, 2013). According to international studies, handwriting is responsible for the variation in the quality of textbooks, since the first year of elementary school (Graham, Berninger, Abbott, & Whitacker, 1997) until undergraduate students (Peverly, 2006).

The quality of manual writing plays a fundamental role in the school performance, since in Brazil the students' academic knowledge, from elementary to high school, are measured through tests which involve proficient writing, either by the bimonthly tests or by the National High School Exam (Enem). However, poor handwriting may mask a student's academic ability, since teachers tend to score higher grades for written tasks, in readable letters than for tasks with illegible letters (McCarney et al., 2013).

When the student is proficient in other areas such as reading and/or mathematics, issues of difficulty with manual writing can be attributed to laziness or lack of motivation, but this may be a misconception, since they can be considered as a specific learning difficulty which affects the production of the language written form (Berninger, Abbott, Augsburger, & Garcia, 2009).

Different researches have been developed to demonstrate differences in gender between students' academic performance in basic areas, such as reading, writing and mathematics. According to the study by Marks (2008), there is a difference in favor of girls towards reading assessments, but in favor of boys concerning math measures. The study by Gibb, Fergusson and Horwood (2008), reports a feminine advantage in all academic areas that arise around the age of 8 and continue until the age of 25. Klecker (2006), supports this feminine advantage in reading, word recognition, and textual comprehension, and Camarata and Woodcock (2005) add reading and writing fluency to girls. There are also studies pointing out that boys' writing differs from girls, so that examiners, such as teachers, would be able to discriminate the gender only by observing the handwriting (Hamid & Loewenthal, 1996; Hanusiak, Oliveira, Justino, & Sabourin, 2012; Hayes, 1996; Sokic, Salihbegovic, & Ahic-Djokic, 2012).

However, when writing legibility interferes in the comprehension of the read material, such as changes in the quality of the letter formation, the alignment and spacing of letters and words, the sizing of letters, among others, there may be indication that the student presents Dysgraphia (Shen, Lee, & Chen, 2012) or, as conceptualized by the DSM-5, "specific learning disorder concerning written disability" (American Psychiatric Association, [APA] 2013). Studies show that dysgraphia may be present in both genders, with or without learning difficulties, learning disorder and dyslexia (Cardoso & Capellini, 2016; Martins et al., 2013,

Mogasale, Patil, Patil & Mogasale 2012; Sumner, Connelly, & Barnett, 2012).

In Brazil, there are a few researches that investigates calligraphy comparing boys and girls, making it difficult to establish the calligraphic profile of the students and, consequently, the investigation of difficulties related to manual writing. Thinking about this and based on the above, this study starts from the hypothesis that there is a relationship between the quality of writing and the gender of elementary school students II. In order to investigate this hypothesis, the following objectives are presented: (1) To verify if there are differences between boys and girls on the evaluation of the quality of the written expression of elementary school students II. (2) To verify if there is gender prevalence in relation to the diagnosis of dysgraphia.

MATERIAL AND METHOD

In order to develop this study, the project was preliminarily evaluated by the Research Ethics Committee of the Faculty of Philosophy and Sciences of the São Paulo State University "Júlio de Mesquita Filho" (FFC/UNESP-Marília-SP) number 0149/2011.

Subjects

A total of 96 students, 41 males (42.7) and 55 females (57.3%) were enrolled in the study, aged from 11 to 14 years and 11 months, from the sixth to the ninth year of elementary school II of a public school of a city in the interior of the State of São Paulo. The students were divided according to their respective school levels (Table 1):

Table 1. Distribution of schoolchildren according to school grade

Distribution of schoolchildren					
School grade	N	Male	%	Female	%
6th grade	27	15	55.6	12	44.4
7th grade	13	6	46.2	7	53.8
8th grade	33	14	42.4	19	57.6
9th grade	23	6	26.1	17	73.9
Total	96	41	42.7	55	57.3

All the students who were present on the day of collection and had delivered the free and informed consent form previously signed by the parents and/or guardians, participated in the study. The students who did not want to participate in the study, and did not bring the signed document, and presented school records related to auditory, visual, motor or intellectual deficiency, or had undergone some intervention (clinical and/or pedagogical) with focus on calligraphy, were excluded from the sample.

Methodological Procedures

Data collection was performed on a single day, inside the room, with the presence of the teacher and the researcher, not exceeding 20 minutes of activity. As a procedure, the Scale of Dysgraphia (Lorenzini, 1993) was used, which consists of the copy of a message (delivered for each student, individually), on an unpublished sheet, using black pencil n ° 2, and without determining enough time for this task (therefore, it does not evaluate writing speed).

This instrument enables the verification of 10 aspects of the handwriting, so that each item of this Scale is punctuated from 0 to 3 points, thus, when the sum of points is equal or superior to eight points and a half, which is equivalent to 50% of the maximum mark (17 marks), writing is considered disgraphic. As follows:

1) floating lines,
2) descending and/or ascending lines,
3) irregular space between words,
4) retouched letters,
5) curvatures and angulations of the arches of "m," "n," "u" and "v,"
6) junction points,
7) collisions and adhesions,
8) jerky movements,
9) irregularity of size and
10) malformed

Statistical Methodology

The data of this research were statistically analyzed by SPSS (Statistical Package for Social Sciences), version 20.0, Minitab 16 and Excel Office 2010. The level of significance (p) 0.05 (5%), that is, all the confidence intervals constructed throughout the work had 95% of statistical confidence.

Parametric statistical tests were used, since the data are quantitative and continuous. In addition, the sample comprises more than 30 subjects, thus, by the Central Limit Theorem, it guarantees that the distribution tends to be Normal.

To make the comparison between boys and girls, in each of the school years, due to the scores obtained in the Scale of dysgraphia, the ANOVA test was employed, which consists of a very usual parametric test, with the purpose of comparing the means of the groups using the variance.

In order to compare the genders on the distribution of the Classification for "Disgraphic," the Equality of Two Proportions test was used, to compare if the proportion of responses of two determined variables and/or their levels are statistically significant.

RESULTS

In response to the first objective, to verify if there are differences between boys and girls in the evaluation of written expression of elementary school students II, based on the ten items assessed by the Dysgraphia scale, there was no statistically significant difference for the items Retouched letters (RL), Junction Points (JP) and Dimensional Irregularity (DI) evidencing that even boys presenting higher prevalence on these items than girls, the performance was similar between them. Although it was identified the item Descendant and Ascendant lines (D/AL) just in writing of the sixth grade students, with prevalence of boys no difference in performance was observed between the genders (Figure 1).

In all the other items assessed by the Dysgraphia Scale, scores were higher for male students with statistically significant difference, in at least one of the school grades (Figure 2).

As for the sum of the 10 items evaluated in the Dysgraphia Scale, it can be observed once again that boys present more dysgraphic manifestations than girls of elementary school II, since for all school years a statistically significant difference was identified in the comparison between them.

D/AL		Media	SD	CV	N	IC	P-valor
6th grade	Fem	0,13	0,23	181%	12	0,13	0,147
	Male	0,27	0,26	97%	15	0,13	
7th grade	Fem	0,00	0,00	- x -	7	- x -	- x -
	Male	0,00	0,00	- x -	6	- x -	
8th grade	Fem	0,00	0,00	- x -	19	- x -	- x -
	Male	0,00	0,00	- x -	14	- x -	
9th grade	Fem	0,00	0,00	- x -	17	- x -	- x -
	Male	0,00	0,00	- x -	6	- x -	

RL		Media	SD	CV	N	IC	P-valor
6th grade	Fem	0,46	0,66	143%	12	0,37	0,252
	Male	0,80	0,82	102%	15	0,41	
7th grade	Fem	0,43	0,79	184%	7	0,58	0,246
	Male	1,00	0,89	89%	6	0,72	
8th grade	Fem	0,47	0,70	147%	19	0,31	0,115
	Male	0,93	0,92	99%	14	0,48	
9th grade	Fem	0,65	0,61	94%	17	0,29	0,104
	Male	1,17	0,75	65%	6	0,60	

JP		Media	SD	CV	N	IC	P-valor
6th grade	Fem	0,17	0,39	234%	12	0,22	0,833
	Male	0,20	0,41	207%	15	0,21	
7th grade	Fem	0,00	0,00	- x -	7	- x -	0,300
	Male	0,17	0,41	245%	6	0,33	
8th grade	Fem	0,00	0,00	- x -	19	- x -	- x -
	Male	0,00	0,00	- x -	14	- x -	
9th grade	Fem	0,06	0,24	412%	17	0,12	0,443
	Male	0,17	0,41	245%	6	0,33	

DI		Media	SD	CV	N	IC	P-valor
6th grade	Fem	0,42	0,51	124%	12	0,29	0,933
	Male	0,40	0,51	127%	15	0,26	
7th grade	Fem	0,00	0,00	- x -	7	- x -	0,300
	Male	0,33	0,82	245%	6	0,65	
8th grade	Fem	0,00	0,00	- x -	19	- x -	0,095
	Male	0,29	0,73	254%	14	0,38	
9th grade	Fem	0,06	0,24	412%	17	0,12	0,443
	Male	0,17	0,41	245%	6	0,33	

Figure 1. Items of the Scale of Dysgraphia that did not show different regarding the sexual gender of elementary school students II.

FL		Media	SD	CV	N	IC	P-valor
6th grade	Fem	0,50	0,52	104%	12	0,30	0,022*
	Male	1,00	0,53	53%	15	0,27	
7th grade	Fem	0,29	0,49	171%	7	0,36	0,005*
	Male	1,17	0,41	35%	6	0,33	
8th grade	Fem	0,58	0,51	88%	19	0,23	0,493
	Male	0,71	0,61	86%	14	0,32	
9th grade	Fem	0,53	0,62	118%	17	0,30	0,499
	Male	0,33	0,52	155%	6	0,41	

ISBW		Media	SD	CV	N	IC	P-valor
6th grade	Fem	0,29	0,33	115%	12	0,19	0,015*
	Male	0,60	0,28	47%	15	0,14	
7th grade	Fem	0,14	0,24	171%	7	0,18	0,053
	Male	0,42	0,20	49%	6	0,16	
8th grade	Fem	0,34	0,24	70%	19	0,11	0,533
	Male	0,39	0,21	54%	14	0,11	
9th grade	Fem	0,32	0,25	76%	17	0,12	0,935
	Male	0,33	0,26	77%	6	0,21	

C/A		Media	SD	CV	N	IC	P-valor
6th grade	Fem	0,08	0,29	346%	12	0,16	0,520
	Male	0,20	0,56	280%	15	0,28	
7th grade	Fem	0,00	0,00	- x -	7	- x -	0,300
	Male	0,08	0,20	245%	6	0,16	
8th grade	Fem	0,08	0,19	237%	19	0,08	0,035*
	Male	0,25	0,26	104%	14	0,14	
9th grade	Fem	0,03	0,12	412%	17	0,06	0,013*
	Male	0,25	0,27	110%	6	0,22	

CA		Media	SD	CV	N	IC	P-valor
6th grade	Fem	1,21	0,75	62%	12	0,43	0,012*
	Male	1,77	0,26	15%	15	0,13	
7th grade	Fem	0,21	0,57	265%	7	0,42	0,052
	Male	1,08	0,86	79%	6	0,69	
8th grade	Fem	0,63	0,76	120%	19	0,34	0,583
	Male	0,79	0,83	105%	14	0,43	
9th grade	Fem	0,26	0,59	223%	17	0,28	0,024*
	Male	1,00	0,77	77%	6	0,62	

SM		Media	SD	CV	N	IC	P-valor
6th grade	Fem	1,08	0,51	48%	12	0,29	0,496
	Male	0,93	0,59	64%	15	0,30	
7th grade	Fem	0,14	0,38	265%	7	0,28	0,155
	Male	0,67	0,82	122%	6	0,65	
8th grade	Fem	0,00	0,00	- x -	19	- x -	0,043*
	Male	0,32	0,67	208%	14	0,35	
9th grade	Fem	0,06	0,24	412%	17	0,12	<0,001*
	Male	0,83	0,41	49%	6	0,33	

MF		Media	SD	CV	N	IC	P-valor
6th grade	Fem	0,00	0,00	- x -	12	- x -	0,108
	Male	0,10	0,21	207%	15	0,10	
7th grade	Fem	0,00	0,00	- x -	7	- x -	0,139
	Male	0,25	0,42	167%	6	0,33	
8th grade	Fem	0,11	0,21	199%	19	0,09	0,012*
	Male	0,39	0,40	102%	14	0,21	
9th grade	Fem	0,03	0,12	412%	17	0,06	<0,001*
	Male	0,67	0,41	61%	6	0,33	

Figure 2. Items of the Dysgraphia Scale that were different regarding the sexual gender of elementary school students II.

Table 2. Comparison of genders regarding performance in the Dysgraphia Scale

Total		Media	Standard deviation	CV	N	IC	P-Valor
6th grade	Female	4.33	1.50	35%	12	0.85	0.006*
	Male	6.27	1.75	28%	15	0.89	
7th grade	Female	1.21	1.63	134%	7	1.21	0.036*
	Male	5.17	4.03	78%	6	3.23	
8th grade	Female	2.05	1.33	65%	19	0.60	0.014*
	Male	4.00	2.87	72%	14	1.50	
9th grade	Female	2.00	1.51	76%	17	0.72	0.001*
	Male	4.92	1.88	38%	6	1.51	

Table 3. Comparison of gender in the diagnosis of dysgraphia

Disgraphic	Female		Male		P-valor
	N	%	N	%	
6th grade	0	0.0%	2	13.3%	0.189
7th grade	0	0.0%	1	16.7%	0.261
8th grade	0	0.0%	2	14.3%	0.089
9th grade	0	0.0%	0	0.0%	- x -

In response to the second objective - to verify if there is prevalence of gender in relation to the diagnosis of dysgraphia - it was observed that only the boys presented a score compatible to dysgraphia, but no statistically significant difference was found in the comparison between genders, characterizing similar performance between boys and girls.

DISCUSSION

The results found in this research showed that there are differences in the quality of the handwriting of elementary school students II when boys and girls are compared. From the 10 items evaluated by the Dysgraphic scale, in six items (floating lines (FL), irregular space between the words (ISBW), curvatures and angulations of the arcades of "m," "n," "u" and "v" (C/A), collisions and adhesions (CA), sudden movements (SM) and malformed (MF) and summing all items, male students presented inferior performance when compared to female students, corroborating findings from other studies (Kim, Al Otaiba, Wanzek, & Gatlin, 2014; Reynolds, Scheiber, Hajovsky, Schwartz, & Kaufman, 2015; Kim, Al Otaiba, & Wanzek, 2015).

According to the literature (Burr, 2002; Hartley, 1991) the quality of writing differs, so that female writing is characterized by being uniform, well organized, with rounded, small and symmetrical letters, while the masculine is rapidly writen, unequal, messy and with pointed and inclined letters. This difference is based on girls' favorable performance regarding language use (Maccoby & Jacklin, 1974; Kim et al., 2015), attitudes toward writing (Knudson, 1995), motivation and self-efficacy (Klassen, 2002; Meece, Glienke, & Burg, 2006), teachers' perceptions (Jones & Myhill, 2004) and individual differences in cognitive abilities, subjacent to writing, such as attention, visual working memory, visual-motor integration, fine motor skills, among others (Bumin & Kavak, 2008; Adams, Simmons, & Willis, 2015).

In order to master writing and use it effectively, writers need to manage several processes that can be characterized as low or high level (Fayol, 1999; Olive, 2014). One of the low-level processes which need to be mastered since the beginning of schooling, consists on transcription, that is, the externalization of the language as written text, which involves the retrieval, assembly and selection of orthographic symbols (ie spelling) and the execution of the motor movements required by a specific writing tool to produce these symbols (ie, handwriting/typing) (Abbott & Berninger, 1993). According to McCutchen (1996), girls tend to automate lower-level transcription skills sooner or more effectively than boys, allowing them to focus on high-order composition skills, while boys still need to consciously focus on the mechanism of writing (Daly, 2003).

Another important point to be highlighted in this study consists on the lack of an item on the dysgraphical scale that has been evidenced in all school years, on the contrary, the items investigated was different for each school grade. This finding is in agreement with the studies of Stainthorp and Rauf (2009) and Berninger and Fuller (1992), who also found gender differences in writing quality, but reported that there is an inconsistent pattern of writing development when the age and gender of the student is taking into account. This inconsistency in writing development can be justified by the associations between memory and writing, since they may vary according to the writer's age, ability, and gender (Bourdieu & Fayol, 1994, Adams, Simmons, & Willis, 2015).

Although no statistically significant difference was found when verifying gender prevalence regarding dysgraphia, the results of this study suggest that boys tend to present the diagnosis. Taking into account that the literature points out a proportion of 2 males: 1 female (Rubin &

Henderson, 1982), and this study found two students in the 6th grade, one in the 7th and two in the 8th year, it is believed that when increasing the sample of students, it becomes possible to confirm this proportion.

It should be highlighted, that even when students grow older and schooling years are advanced, the quality of handwriting continues to be an essential factor for the composition of texts (Olive, Favart, Beauvais, & Beauvais, 2009) and this ability is positively associated with other academic skills (Wollscheid, Sjaastad, & Tømte, 2016). Therefore, educational professionals should be aware of the importance of teaching, not only handwriting skills in the early years, but they should also practice these skills during subsequent school years, taking into account the differences between genders throughout the writing process.

Conclusion

The results presented in this study showed that boys tend to present greater difficulties regarding handwriting when compared to elementary school girls II. And, although no statistically significant difference was found regarding dysgraphia, it was possible to identify only boys with the diagnosis.

Based on these findings, handwriting cannot be overlooked and deserves more attention from professionals in the area of education, since male and female students behave differently during process of developing this ability.

Aware of the limitations of this study, new investigations are necessary with the inclusion of instruments capable of evaluating the cognitive abilities underlying writing, such as: visual work memory, visual perception and attention, aiming to relate them to the calligraphy of Brazilian male and female students.

ACKNOWLEDGMENT

We are grateful to Capes (Coordination for the Improvement of Higher Education Personnel) for the PhD scholarship granted to the first author.

REFERENCES

Abbott, R. D., & Berninger, V. W. (1993). Structural equation modeling of relationships among developmental skills and writing skills in primary- and intermediate-grade writers. *Journal of Educational Psychology*, 85(3), 478-508. doi:10.1037/0022-0663.85.3.478.

Adams, A.-M., Simmons, F., & Willis, C. (2015). Exploring relationships between working memory and writing: individual differences associated with gender. *Learning and Individual Differences*, 40, 101-107. doi:10.1016/j.lindif.2015.04.011.

American Psychiatric Association. (2013). *Diagnostic and statistical manual of mental health disorders*. (5th ed.). Arlington, VA: American Psychiatric Publishing.

Berninger, V. W., Abbott, R. D., Augsburger, A., & Garcia, N. (2009). Comparison of pen and keyboard transcription modes in children with and without learning disabilities. *Learning Disability Quarterly*, 32(3), 123-141. doi:10.2307/27740364.

Berninger, V. W., & Fuller, F. (1992). Gender differences in orthographic, verbal, and compositional fluency: implications for assessing writing disabilities in primary grade children. *Journal of School Psychology*, 30(4), 363-382. doi:10.1016/0022-4405(92)90004-0.

Bourdin, B., & Fayol, M. (1994). Is written language production more difficult than oral language production? A working memory approach. *International Journal of Psychology*, 29(5), 591-620. doi:10.1080/00207599408248175.

Bumin, G., & Kavak, S. T. (2008). An investigation of the factors affecting handwriting performance in children with hemiplegic cerebral palsy. *Disability and Rehabilitation*, 30(18), 1374-1385.

Burr, V. (2002). Judging gender from samples of adult handwriting: accuracy and use of cues. *The Journal of Social Psychology*, 142(6), 691-700.

Camarata, S., & Woodcock, R. (2005). Sex differences in processing speed: developmental effects in males and females. *Intelligence*, 34(3), 231-252. doi:10.1016/j.intell.2005.12.001.

Cardoso, M. H., & Capellini, S. A. (2016). Identificação e caracterização da disgrafia em escolares com dificuldades e transtornos de aprendizagem. *Distúrbios da Comunicação* [Identification and characterization of dysgraphia in schoolchildren with learning difficulties and disorders. *Communication Disorders*], 28(1), 27-37. Disponível em: https://revistas.pucsp.br/index.php/dic/article/view/23948/19268.

Daly, C. (2003). *Yes he can — Schools where boys write well.* London: Ofsted.

Fayol, M. (1999). From on-line management problems to strategies in written composition. In M. Torrance, & G. Jeffery (Eds.). *The cognitive demands of writing: processing capacity and working memory effects in text production* (pp. 13-23). Amsterdam: Amsterdam University Press.

Gibb, S. J., Fergusson, D. M., & Horwood, L. J. (2008). Gender differences in educational achievement to age 25. *Australian Journal of Education*, 52(1), 63-80. doi:10.1177/000494410805200105.

Graham, S., Berninger, V. W., Abbot, R. D., Abbot, S. P., & Whitaker, D. (1997). Role of mechanics in composing of elementary school students: a new methodological approach. *Journal of Educational Psychology*, 89(1), 170-182. doi:10.1037/0022-0663.89.1.170.

Hamid, S., & Loewenthal, K. M. (1996). Inferring gender from handwriting in Urdu and English. *The Journal of Social Psychology*, 136(6), 778-782.

Hanusiak, R. K., Oliveira, L. S., Justino, E., & Sabourin, R. (2012). Writer verification using texture-based features. *International Journal on Document Analysis and Recognition*, 15(3), 213-226. doi:10.1007/s10032-011-0166-4.

Hartley, J. (1991). Sex differences in handwriting: a comment on spear. *British Educational Research Journal*, 17(2), 141-145.

Hayes, W. N. (1996). Identifying sex from handwriting. *Perceptual Motor Skills*, 83(3), 791-800.

Jones, S., & Myhill, D. (2004). 'Troublesome boys' and 'compliant girls': Gender identity and perceptions of achievement and underachievement. *British Journal of Sociology of Education*, 25(5), 547-561.

Kim, Y. S., Al Otaiba, S., & Wanzek, J. (2015). Kindergarten predictors of third grade writing. *Learning and Individual Differences*, 37, 27-37. doi:10.1016/j.lindif.2014.11.009.

Kim, Y.-S., Al Otaiba, S., Wanzek, J., & Gatlin, B. (2014). Toward an understanding of dimensions, predictors, and the gender gap in written composition. *Journal of Educational Psychology*, 107(1), 79-95. doi:10.1037/a0037210.

Klassen, R. (2002). Writing in early adolescence: a review of the role of self-efficacy beliefs. *Educational Psychology Review*, 14(2), 173-203.

Klecker, B. M. (2006). The gender gap in NAEP fourth-, eighth-, and twelfth-grade reading scores across years. *Reading Improvement*, 43(1), 50-56.

Knudson, R. E. (1995). Writing experiences, attitudes and achievement of first to sixth graders. *The Journal of Educational Research*, 89(2), 90-97.

Lorenzini, M. V. (1993). *Uma escala para detectar a disgrafia baseada na escala de Ajuriaguerra* [*A scale for detecting dysgraphia based on the Ajuriaguerra scale*]. (Dissertação de mestrado não publicada). Universidade Federal de São Carlos, São Carlos, SP.

Maccoby, E. E., & Jacklin, C. N. (1974). *The psychology of sex differences*. Stanford, CA: Stanford University Press.

Marks, G. N. (2008). Accounting for the gender gaps in student performance in reading and mathematics: evidence from 31 countries. *Oxford Review of Education*, 34(1), 89-109. doi:10.1080/03054980701565279.

Martins, M. R. I., Bastos, J. A., Cecato, A. T., Araujo, M. L. S., Magro, R. R., & Alaminos, V. (2013). Screening for motor dysgraphia in public schools. *Jornal de Pediatria*, 89(1), 70-74. doi:10.1016/j.jped.2013.02.011.

McCarney, D., Peters, L., Jackson, S., Thomas, M., & Kirby, A. (2013). Does poor handwriting conceal literacy potential in primary school children? *International Journal of Disability, Development and Education*, 60(2), 105-118. doi:10.1080/1034912X.2013.786561.

McCutchen, D. (1996). A capacity theory of writing: working memory in composition. *Educational Psychology Review*, 8(3), 299-325.

Meece, J. L., Glienke, B. B., & Burg, S. (2006). Gender and motivation. *Journal of School Psychology*, 44(5), 351-373. doi:10.1016/j.jsp.2006.04.004.

Mogasale, V. V., Patil, V. D., Patil, N. M., & Mogasale, V. (2012). Prevalence of specific learning disabilities among primary school children in a South Indian city. *Indian Journal of Pediatrics*, 79(3), 342-347. doi:10.1007/s12098-011-0553-3.

Olive, T., Favart, M., Beauvais, C., & Beauvais, L. (2009). Children's cognitive effort and fluency in writing: effects of genre and of handwriting automatization. *Learning and Instruction*, 19(4), 299-308. doi:10.1016/j.learninstruc.2008. 05.005.

Olive, T. (2014). Toward a parallel and cascading model of thewriting system: a review of research on writing processes coordination. *Journal of Writing Research*, 6(2), 173-194. doi:10.17239/jowr-2014.06.02.4.

Peverly, S. T. (2006). The importance of handwriting speed in adult writing. *Developmental Neuropsychology*, 29(1), 197-216. doi:10.1207/s15326942dn2901_10.

Reynolds, M. R., Scheiber, C., Hajovsky, D. B., Schwartz, B., & Kaufman, A. S. (2015). Gender differences in academic achievement: is writing an exception to the gender similarities hypothesis? *The Journal of Genetic Psychology: Research and Theory on Human Development*, 176(4), 211-234. doi:10.1080/00221325.2015.1036833.

Rubin, N., & Henderson, S. E. (1982). Two sides of the same coin: variation in 33 teaching methods and failure to learn to write. *British Journal of Special Education*, 9(4), 17-24. doi:10.1111/j.1467-8578.1982.tb00576.x.

Shen, I.-H., Lee, T.-Y., & Chen, C.-L. (2012). Handwriting performance and underlying factors in children with Attention Deficit Hyperactivity Disorder. *Research in Developmental Disabilities*, 33(4), 1301-1309. doi:10.1016/j.ridd.2012.02.010.

Sokic, E., Salihbegovic, A., & Ahic-Djokic, M. (2012). Analysis of offline handwritten text samples of different gender using shape descriptors. In *Proceedings of IX International Symposium on Telecommunications (BIHTEL)*, (pp. 1-6). Sarajevo, Bosnia & Herzegovina: IEEE. doi:10.1109/BIHTEL.2012.6412086.

Stainthorp, R., & Rauf, N. (2009). An investigation of the influence of the transcription skills of handwriting and spelling on the quality of text writing by girls and boys in Key Stage 2. *Handwriting Today*, 8, 9-13.

Sumner, E., Connelly, V., & Barnett, A. (2012). Children with dyslexia are slow writers because they pause more often and not because they are slow at handwriting execution. *Reading & Writing*, 26(6), 991-1008. doi:10.1007/s11145-012-9403-6.

Wollscheid, S., Sjaastad, J., & Tømte, C. (2016). The impact of digital devices vs. Pen(cil) and paper on primary school students' writing skills: a research review. *Computers & Education*, 95, 19-35. doi:10.1016/j.compedu.2015.12.001.

In: Handwriting and Dysgrafia
Editors: M. Herrera Cardoso et al.
ISBN: 978-1-53613-805-4

Chapter 7

HANDWRITING AND ORTHOGRAPHIC LEARNING

***Esmeralda Sandra Santos Damasceno*[1,*], *Mirian Aratangy Arnaut*[1], *Valéria de Cássia Marques*[1] *and Clara Regina Brandão de Avila*[1,2]**

[1]Graduate Program in Human Communication Disorders – Federal University of São Paulo (UNIFESP), São Paulo, Brazil

[2]Department of Speech Therapy, São Paulo School of Medicine – Federal University of São Paulo (UNIFESP), São Paulo, Brazil

ABSTRACT

Changes in the shaping of letters can be related to the frequency of writing errors. Through the analysis of a sample of 80 schoolchildren handwriting from the second to the fifth year of primary/junior high schools, from both the public and private networks of the city of São Paulo, it was sought to identify whether changes in the shaping of the letter could increase the number of orthographic errors. The children were recommended by their teachers as they performed well at school. The

[*] Corresponding Author: hesksandra@gmail.com

following items were selected from Lorenzini's Dysgraphia Scale: junction points; collisions and adhesions, irregularities in size, and poorly formed letters, in order to define groups based on the presence or absence of these irregularities. The errors in writing were classified according to their orthographic character. Performance was compared by school year and correlations were investigated. Statistical tests and level of significance for values of $p < 0.05$ evidenced differences in the quantity of errors according to the presence of irregularities in the shaping of letters, mainly in the private schools.

Keywords: handwriting, evaluation, specific learning disorders, spelling

INTRODUCTION

Writing is a human invention, created to represent ideas, feelings and thoughts. Its learning, undertaken through formal instruction, is most intense during the first three years of school (National Common Curricular Basis, 2016) and, like any learning process, depends on encouragement from external agents (physical, social, etc.), on the maturation of the Central Nervous System, and on cognitive development. There are two main components in learning handwriting: graphmotor and orthographic skills. The ability to write by hand involves sensory-motor, kinesthetic and cognitive information.

One of the motor components in handwriting is the same one responsible for maintaining the child's posture. General posture is important during the specific gripping and correct handling of the instrument for carrying out the shaping which results in the appropriate writing of each letter and word on the paper (Dias & Avila, 2008). Intelligence, attention and memory are abilities which allow the selective sensory capture (visual) of the shapes and the spatial guidance of the letter to be copied or written.

The orthographic learning depends on the development of certain language skills. From early childhood, the child receives linguistic encouragement and has specific experiences for developing oral language, above all involving observation in the use of speech sounds until she masters the rules of using phonemes. In the preschool phase, the child is able to think objectively about the knowledge that she has of words, plays with rhymes and speech sounds, and begins the process of formal knowledge of letters, leading to activities which permit her to master the alphabetic principle for coding and decoding writing. Information on correct writing becomes known, through reading, and is meta-analyzed with the support of morphosyntactic knowledge. This allows the system of orthographic rules to be grasped and applied during graphic expression. Fine motor control is an indispensable skill for undertaking actions which require dexterity – in this case, the precise shaping of the letters (Rosenblum, Aloni, & Josman, 2010; Okuda, Lourencetti, Santos, Padula, & Capellini, 2011).

The learning of writing depends, therefore, on a formal teaching process (letter-sound association), and on the dexterity needed to form the letter shape. Learning to shape each letter in order to connect them to form words requires, therefore, neurological maturation and consequent development of specific skills. The association of the letter shape with the phoneme allows the child to make choices and adjustments and to select from a repertoire of codes either already learned or in a process of learning – as well as the effectiveness and recovery of these records in the form of letters and numbers. The experience of the repetitive undertaking of letters is recorded in the motor and cognitive areas of the Central Nervous System (CNS) whose synaptic circuitry works automatically for the writing of already-known forms and serves as a basic model for the learning of new formats (Rotta, Ohweiler, & Riesgo, 2015).

Different processes are triggered when writing by hand. In dictation or free production tasks, for example, the evocation of the word is triggered and requires the selection of graphemes. It is important to remember that psycholinguistic characteristics, such as extension, familiarity and orthographic regularity (Lambert, Alamargot, Larocque, & Caporossi, 2011) interfere in this process, which depends, from the collective point of view, on the structure of the orthographic system of the language and, from the point of view of the individual, on attention and on operational and long-term memory, in order to resolve the orthographic difficulty. Pauses and erasures are often observed during this process, which follows the identification of the letter (which must become automatic during the first years of school education) under the influence of the form characteristics required for each letter, and of the need to connect, sequentially, different letters that make up the word – and to recognize spatial limits between different words which make up the sentence (Van Galen, Meulenbroek & Hylkema, 1986). Visual fixation and visual tracking accompany this whole process. This axis of development can raise concerns regarding mastering graphomotor skills and the orthographic knowledge, when difficulties in writing correctly are manifested or continue throughout the child's years at school – as, in order to communicate ideas, a person's handwriting must be legible, spatially organized, and obey the orthographic conventions of the language's system (Gombert, 2009).

Writing, as a significant communicative activity, must associate handwritten form with meaning - form with content. During the learning of the alphabetical principle, the language's rules and grammatical and orthographic conventions are grasped, and the establishing of rules for spacing and separation of the letters ensures the legibility which allows the desired transmission of information. As a result, the handwriting regularity and accuracy, the letters and words organization in the space and the time spent in carrying out the task are characteristics which promote legibility. The automaticity of writing, with good legibility and appropriate speed, allows the child to direct her attention to the word's composition in its phonological and orthographic characteristics. This skill must facilitate self-monitoring and self-correction, promoting the learning of orthographically correct writing.

Difficulties in fine motor coordination can hinder the learning of writing by hand legibly, with consequences for orthographic learning – although this also depends on reading and on good conditions for processing phonological, morphosyntactic and orthographic information (Okuda et al., 2011; Guimarães & Paula, 2010). For Zesiger, Deonnae and Mayor (2000), it is at the age of approximately 12 years old that the student acquires speed, fluidity and regularity in writing.

The literature has evidenced the presence of correlations between handwriting and spelling characteristics (Feder & Majnemer, 2007; Okuda et al., 2011), whether in normal or in altered development. Besides this, in a significant percentage of people, two different situations of irregularities in writing – dysorthography (ICD 10 – F81.1) and dysgraphia – accompany, together, many cases of dyslexia (Capellini, Coppede & Valle, 2010).

In dysorthography, one can observe the incorrect writing of words; in dysgraphia, there is impairment in the undertaking of the format of the letters, with mixing of upper and lowercase letters, mixing of block and cursive letters, and unintelligible and/or incomplete format of the letters. In both conditions, one can observe changes in the written expression, with impairment of skills such as: automatically identifying words and writing without changes to what has been handwritten, writing without swapping letters, without inappropriately joining or separating the words, without confusing syllables, without omitting letters and inversions, without changes in the format of the letter and without spacing, besides perceiving the graphic indications such as paragraphs, accentuation and punctuation (Gombert,2009; Nicolson & Fawcett, 2011). These alterations can have a psychosocial impact on the development of students who present them. Between 10 and 30% of the school population are dysgraphic (Kushki, Schwellnus, Iliyas, & Chau, 2011).

Some studies have investigated handwriting characteristics and the use of orthographic rules in different learning conditions. One study on dysgraphia (Oliveira, 2000) analyzed the handwriting of children enrolled in the public and private education systems, both with and without writing difficulties, and from different socioeconomic levels. Results indicated that family income was relevant in the prevalence of dysgraphia, and suggested that in families with lower purchasing power, the use of writing and its encouragement are restricted.

The other type of writing problem – dysorthography – is also studied, perhaps with even greater concern, as, in these cases, the objective is to seek and understand the relationship between writing errors and: the level of metacognitive development (Maluf, 2003; Veloso, 2003; Nobile &

Barrera, 2009); oral language performance; auditory perception; and the orthographic processing and learning. The spelling should reveal all of these skills.

Different studies undertaken with Brazilian schoolchildren have shown that the learning of writing in Portuguese – despite being a language reasonably transparent in orthographic terms – is a process which predicts the appearance of errors whose frequency, defined by their orthographic complexity, is expected to be reduced as the child's schooling progresses, until it finally disappears (Rosenblum et al., 2010; Zorzi & Ciasca, 2008; Gonçalves & Capellini, 2010). Less importance, however, is given to issues related to the accuracy of the handwriting and to the possibility of there being an association between this and the orthographic error. As noted, the learning of the correct writing also depends on self-correction. It is therefore fair to ask whether difficulty in letter forming can hinder this process of self-learning. The literature indicates that the child who still needs to concentrate her attention in order to think how to shape a letter may present impairment in the writing legibility, and – consequently – in the quality of the content and in her orthographic self-monitoring and self-correction capacity (Jones & Christensen, 1999), although these skills develop more significantly after the beginning of adolescence.

The majority of studies on the characterization of orthographic errors in children, with different learning problems, have observed the presence of subjects with dysgraphia and many types of orthographic error, the most recurrent type being the multiple representations (Zorzi & Ciasca, 2008; Arnaut, Avila & Hackerott, 2010; Arnaut, 2015). One recent study identified correlations between irregularities in the letter format and a greater number of writing errors of a phonological character (Damasceno, Avila & Arnaut, 2015).

The presentation which follows in this chapter will show evidence that children with irregularities in the letter format can present a greater number of orthographic errors. The authors sought to differentiate groups of students from primary school, by the characteristics of the shaping of letters, the frequency of the occurrence of errors with an orthographic character, and by whether they were educated publicly or privately.

Although samples of writing of noun phrases were studied, the analyses focused on investigating the words, with the objective of identifying whether alterations in the letter shaping could differentiate the students writing with a higher or lower number of errors with an orthographic character.

METHOD

This chapter shows a retrospective, transversal, quantitative analysis study. It was approved by the Research Ethics Committee under N. 1768/11. Consent forms were signed by parents or guardians of all the participants.

A total of eighty samples of writing from dictation of 34 noun phrases were analyzed. These writings were produced by students (53.22% boys) aged between 07 and 11 years old, and enrolled in the 2nd to 5th years of primary school, in public and private schools in the city of São Paulo. All the children were performing well at school (stated by their teachers) and had no complaints or indicators of auditory or (uncorrected) visual disabilities or of neurological, behavioral or cognitive disorders. A total of 20 protocols from each school year were analyzed (10 from the public school network, and 10 from the private school network). Data collection was undertaken during the second trimester of the school year. The noun phrases were written in pencil, on blank, lined paper, with a space of 10 mm between lines. Children were instructed not to erase mistakes; they were to cross out the word and continue writing. The sample was analyzed by a speech therapist who had received instruction in the use of Lorenzini's Dysgraphia Scale (Lorenzini, 2003) applied for analyzing the sample handwriting.

Lorenzini's Dysgraphia Scale is made up of 10 items which allows the analysis of aspects of the handwriting. For this study, which investigated the issue of orthography, at the level of the word, the following items were selected: a) junction point: the child is not able to link the letters together, and raises the pencil or pen from the paper, placing it back in order to rejoin the letters she has just made to that which she had previously made; b) collisions or adhesions: the student squashes one letter over the other, causing an overlapping; c) irregularity in size: improper variation in the size of the letters within long words. The person may write small or large letters, and the proportions of the three zones of writing (upper, middle and lower zones) are not respected; d) poor shapes: letters are made with deformities, which causes the letters' appearance to be unaesthetic and outside, or differing from, the standard. To a certain extent, these items should be sufficient to assess the handwriting at the level of the word – as the junction points, collisions and adhesions can cause the incorrect segmentation and word junction; the irregularity of size and poor shaping can cause difficulty in identifying the written letters, making it hard for the student to be corrected.

The sample of writing was also analyzed by its orthographic characteristics. Only orthographic errors were considered, according to the classification proposed by Arnaut et al., (2010): a) accentuation in the handwriting; b) phonetic interference in spelling resulting from writing as it is spoken (for instance, writing 'blu' instead of 'blue'); c) incorrect use of letters (use of grapheme, according to the context).

The 80 samples of writing were grouped and analyzed according to the frequency of irregularities in the letter shape, as following:

1. Regarding the junction points: G1 - when 04 or fewer junction points were evident; or G2 - when 05 or more junction points were evident.
2. Regarding irregularities in size: G1 - absence of irregularities in size; or G2 - there was variation in dimension in 01 or 03 long words.
3. Regarding the poor shaping of letters: G1 - absence of poor shaping: or G2 - presence of 01 or more badly-shaped letters.
4. Regarding the collisions or adhesions: G1 - absence of collisions and adhesions; G2 - when 01 or more collisions and adhesions were evident.

Although, according to the Lorenzini Dysgraphia Scale, some writings could be classified as dysgraphic, this chapter considers only the absence or presence of irregularities in handwriting. These, and the orthographic errors, were identified and tabulated. The average were calculated for the number of samples (or children) who presented the irregularities sought, by whether they were enrolled in public or private schools.

The Kolmogorov-Smirnov test of normality for samples greater than 30 cases was conducted, and the variables did not follow the standard normal distribution. The nonparametric Mann-Whitney test was indicated to compare two groups (G1 and G2) with a level of numerical measurement and independent samples with non-normal distribution. The level of statistical significance was stipulated for values of $p < 0.05$.

RESULTS

The analysis of the junction point showed, among the students of private schools, that those who presented this irregularity showed more errors of the type involving incorrect use of a letter, and others involving accentuation. The same response profile found in private schools was observed in the public network, with more misuse of letters, although the p value of p (0.062) is marginal, and errors when accenting words with more letter junction points observed.

The analysis of irregularities in size showed – among privately-educated children – that students who presented this irregularity in handwriting presented more errors involving the incorrect use of letters, and errors involving accentuation. Among the children enrolled in public schools, there was no difference between the groups.

The comparison of groups regarding the presence of collisions and adhesions did not evidence differences in the frequency of any type of orthographic errors, and in either private or public education.

Table 1. Comparison of schoolchildren performance without (G1) and with junction points (G2), by educational system (public or private) and type of spelling error

Type of error			Junction points		Mann-Whitney test (p)	Result
			G1	G2		
Private	Incorrect use of a letter	Mean	2.32	4.67	0.015*	1 < 2
		Median	2.00	4.50		
		Standard-deviation	2.30	3.31		
		n	22	18		
	Phonetic interference	Mean	.82	1.33	.062#	1 = 2
		Median	.00	1.00		
		Standard-deviation	1.26	1.03		
		n	22	18		
	Accentuation	Mean	2.09	4.50	0.019*	1 < 2
		Median	1.50	5.00		
		Standard deviation	2.29	3.03		
		n	22	18		
Public	Incorrect use of a letter	Mean	5.40	7.50	.063#	1 = 2
		Median	5.00	7.00		
		Standard-deviation	2.95	3.61		
		n	20	20		
	Phonetic interference	Mean	2.90	3.40	.211	1 = 2
		Median	2.00	3.50		
		Standard-deviation	1.97	1.39		
		n	20	20		
	Accentuation	Mean	5.30	7.15	0.009*	1 < 2
		Median	5.00	7.00		
		Standard-deviation	2.79	2.28		
		n	20	20		

Mann-Whitney test; value of statistical significance fixed at $p < 0.05$; Key: (nearly significant).

Table 2. Comparison of schoolchildren performance, without (G1) and with (G2) irregularities in the size of letters, by education system (publicor private) and type of spelling error

Type of error			Irregularity in size		Mann-Whitney test (p)	Result
			G1	G2		
Private	Incorrect use of a letter	Mean	1.80	4.32	0.015*	1 < 2
		Median	2.00	4.00		
		Standard-deviation	1.47	3.30		
		n	15	25		
	Phonetic interference	Mean	.73	1.24	0.267	1 = 2
		Median	1.00	1.00		
		Standard-deviation	.88	1.30		
		n	15	25		
	Accentuation	Mean	1.27	4.32	0.001*	1 < 2
		Median	1.00	5.00		
		Standard-deviation	1.53	2.91		
		n	15	25		
Public	Incorrect use of a letter	Mean	6.25	6.50	0.753	1 = 2
		Median	5.50	6.00		
		Standard-deviation	4.03	3.32		
		n	8	32		
	Phonetic interference	Mean	3.75	3.00	0.539	1 = 2
		Median	3.50	3.00		
		Standard-deviation	2.49	1.46		
		n	8	32		
	Accentuation	Mean	5.50	6.41	0.584	1 = 2
		Median	6.00	6.00		
		Standard-deviation	2.67	2.70		
		n	8	32		

Mann-Whitney test; value of statistical significance fixed at $p < 0.05$.

Table 3. Comparison of schoolchildren performance without (G1) and with (G2) poor shaping letters, by educationsystem (public/private) and type of spelling error

Type of error			Poorshapes		Mann-Whitney test (p)	Result
			G1	G2		
Private	Incorrect use of a letter	Mean	1.67	3.68		
		Median	1.50	2.00	0.137	1 = 2
		Standard-deviation	1.63	3.10		
		n	6	34		
	Phonetic interference	Mean	.67	1.12		
		Median	.50	1.00	0.493	1 = 2
		Standard-deviation	.82	1.23		
		n	6	34		
	Accentuation	Mean	.83	3.59		
		Median	1.00	3.00	0.030*	1 < 2
		Standard-deviation	.75	2.92		
		n	6	34		
Public	Incorrect use of a letter	Mean	6.60	6.43		
		Median	6.00	6.00	0.937	1 = 2
		Standard-deviation	3.91	3.41		
		n	5	35		
	Phonetic interference	Mean	4.40	2.97		
		Median	4.00	3.00	0.261	1 = 2
		Standard-deviation	2.70	1.48		
		n	5	35		
	Accentuation	Mean	5.80	6.29		
		Median	7.00	6.00	1.000	1 = 2
		Standard-deviation	2.39	2.75		
		n	5	35		

Mann-Whitney test; value of statistical significance fixed at $p < 0.05$.

Table 4. Comparison of schoolchildren performance without (G1) and with (G2) collisions and adhesions, by education system (public/private) and type of spelling error

Type of error			Collisions and adhesions		Mann-Whitney test (p)	Result
			G1	G2		
Private	Incorrect use of a letter	Mean	2.10	3.80	0.246	1 = 2
		Median	2.00	2.50		
		Standard-deviation	1.29	3.29		
		n	10	30		
	Phonetic interference	Mean	.80	1.13	0.469	1 = 2
		Median	.50	1.00		
		Standard-deviation	1.03	1.22		
		n	10	30		
	Accentuation	Mean	1.70	3.67	0.109	1 = 2
		Median	1.50	3.50		
		Standard-deviation	1.83	3.02		
		n	10	30		
Public	Incorrect use of a letter	Mean	6.30	6.50	0.842	1 = 2
		Median	5.50	6.00		
		Standard-deviation	3.06	3.58		
		n	10	30		
	Phonetic interference	Mean	4.00	2.87	0.148	1 = 2
		Median	4.00	2.50		
		Standard-deviation	2.00	1.53		
		n	10	30		
	Accentuation	Mean	6.80	6.03	0.508	1 = 2
		Median	6.50	6.00		
		Standard-deviation	2.97	2.61		
		n	10	30		

Mann-Whitney test; value of statistical significance fixed at $p < 0.05$.

It was only in the private education system that differences between the groups with a greater mean number of errors involving accentuation produced by students who most presented poor format of letters were ascertained.

Comments

Progressive improvement in the handwriting and in the orthographic learning is expected as a consequence of Central Nervous System maturation, and, obviously of the progress of child's education (Zorzi & Ciasca, 2008). The increase in the readability of written production should facilitate the identification of errors, formally indicated, or even during self-correction activities (and consequent self-learning). This graphomotor and visual-perceptive process is, naturally, accompanied by a progressive reduction in the number of orthographic errors (Rosenblum et al., 2010). However, this pattern of development is not always observed. Some schoolchildren seem to take a different path, showing greater diversity and frequency of errors in writing which requires great efforts to be eliminated (Zorzi & Ciasca, 2008).

The hypothesis that characteristics of the letter format may be related to orthographic processing errors, was raised from the clinical observation of schoolchildren writing, and from a previous study results which evidenced associations between these two variables when the error studied was of a phonological nature (Damasceno et al., 2015).

A simple view of the tables show numerically higher average for orthographic errors among the children enrolled in public schools, data which was expected, but not analyzed statistically. Considering these numbers, it is possible to question the teaching quality these children received. The same errors, however, also appeared among the privately-educated children, and some of these were more frequent in G2, when compared with G1. That is to say, in the presence of handwriting, there was a higher number of errors.

In this process of learning to write, the child is expected to completely master the skill of writing legibly by hand. However, in the beginning, it is necessary for an adult to show the schoolchild where to start the shaping of the letter, and the movements necessary for connecting one letter to the next (Zesiger et al., 2000; Rotta et al., 2015). In this chapter, the samples of writing with more than five junction points showed more orthographic errors involving the incorrect use of letters and errors involving accentuation in the writing. This result was the same, regardless of whether the child was in a public or private school. The learning or use of orthographic rules dependent on the context can be impaired when the letters of a single word are separated. Besides, if during the writing, the attention is focused on shaping the letters, the result can be a future impairment of correct writing. The sample also contained the writing of 5th grade children, who were closer to certain handwriting automatisms (Rotta et al., 2015).

When the samples of writing were grouped by characteristics involving irregularities in the size of the letters, the same types of orthographic errors – the incorrect use of letters, or errors involving accentuation – were found in higher numbers in G2 among the children of private schools. Although accentuation of words is related more to phonological issues (identification of tonic syllable), irregularities in the size of letters can hinder the reading of the production itself or the identification of the place where the correction should be made (Van Galen et al., 1986). The absence of difference between G1 and G2 among children enrolled in public schools was accompanied by high error average occurrence averages of the three types considered.

The presence of poor letter shaping evidenced a higher number of accentuation errors in groupG2, but only among children of private schools. The three types of error were present in similar frequencies in the writings which either presented or did not present collisions and adhesions, in both public and private education networks.

Analyzed by type of error, the samples evidenced more errors related to multiple representations and accentuation, which are the last rules to be mastered by Brazilian students. Interference in spelling caused by the child spelling out the word phonetically showed a lower frequency of occurrence in both private and public school. In this analysis, it is necessary to consider that the sample is made up of children from four different school years, without learning problems. Obviously, the eighty participants varied in performance, which may explain the presence of errors associated with the shaping of irregular and inaccurate letters. As a result, it is reasonable to think that the errors found may indeed be characteristic of students with worse performance in writing by hand, in orthography, and in the quality of the orthographic writing. It is necessary to remember that irregularities in the handwriting of the letters which may resemble characteristics of dysgraphia may also be found in students without learning problems, such as those who participated in this study (Rotta et al., 2015; Coppede, Okuda & Capellini., 2012).

Although the participants' motor function was not evaluated, literature indicates that the better the performance of fine and global motor function, the lower will be the frequency of dysgraphia or irregularities in the handwriting of letters (Capellini et al., 2010).

Final Considerations

Statistical limitations were related to the size and distribution of the sample. Even so, it was possible to identify a greater number of orthographic errors in the presence of irregularities in children's handwriting, than in their absence, particularly in private schools. For example, the fact that the child has to complete the connection between the letters of a word, after writing it, showed in a more homogenous way (regarding the private or public school) that a great number of errors, involving the incorrect use of letters and accentuation, may be present when junction points are still necessary. Child's attention, directed towards the letter shape, may impair correct writing, even in children without learning problems. It is, therefore, reasonable to be concerned with the effect of handwriting quality on the learning and use of orthographic rules.

REFERENCES

Arnaut, M. A., Avila, C. R. B. & Hackerott, M. M. S. (2010). Entre a ortografia e a patologia. In *Anais IP:2010, 13º Congresso Brazileiro de Língua Portuguesa* [Between spelling and pathology. In Anais IP: 2010, *13th Brazilian Congress of Portuguese Language*]. São Paulo. PUC-SP.

Arnaut M. A. (2015). *Avaliação da escrita por meio de sintagmas nominais.* (Tese de Doutorado) [*Writing evaluation by means of nominal phrases* (Doctoral thesis)]. UNIFESP. São Paulo – SP.

Base Nacional Comum Curricular – 2ª versão 11/05/2016 Volume 02 [*National Common Curricular Base - 2nd version 05/11/20*16] Volume 02- Língua Portuguesa pág. 187. portal.mec.gov.br › PAR › Secretarias › SEB - Educação Básica acesso em 26/05/2016.

Calvo, A. P. (2007). *A Produção gráfica e escrita focalizando a variação da produção de força dos dedos.* (Dissertação de Mestrado) [*A Graphic and writing production focusing on the variation of finger force production.* (Masters dissertation)]. Universidade Estadual Paulista. Rio Claro – SP.

Capellini, S. A., Coppede, A. C. & Valle, T. R. (2010). Função motora fina de escolares com dislexia, distúrbio e dificuldades de aprendizagem. *Pró-Fono Revista de Atualização Científica* [Fine motor function of schoolchildren with dyslexia, disturbance and learning difficulties. *Pro-Fono Scientific Update Magazine*], *22*(3), 201-208.doi.org/ 10.1590/S0104-56872010000300008.

Coppede, A. C., Okuda, P. M. M., & Capellini, S. A. (2012). Performance of children with learning difficulties in fine motor function and handwriting. *Revista Brazileira de crescimento e desenvolvimento humano,* 22(3), 297-306.

Damasceno, E. S. S., Avila, C. R. B. & Arnaut, M. A. (2015). Correlações entre o traçado da escrita manual e o desempenho Fundamental I. *Revista Distúrbios da Comunicação* [Correlations between manual writing and Fundamental performance I. *Communication Disorders Magazine*], 27(4), 819-830.

Dias, R. S. & Avila, C. R. B. (2008). Uso e conhecimento ortográfico no transtorno específico de leitura. *Revista da Sociedade Brazileira de Fonoaudiologia* [Use and spelling knowledge in specific reading disorder. *Journal of the Brazilian Society of Speech Therapy*], 13(4), 381-90.

Elliott, J. M. & Connolly, K. J. (1984). A classification of manipulative hand movements. *Developmental Medicine & Child Neurology,* 26 (3), 283-96.

Fayol, M. (2013). *L'acquisition de l'écrit. Que sais-je?* [*The acquisition of writing. What do I know?*] Paris:PUF- Presse Universitaire de France.

Feder, K. P. & Majnemer, A. (2007). Handwriting development, competency and intervention. *Developmental Medicine & Child Neurology,* 49(1), 312-7.

Gombert, J. E. (2009). L'apprentissage de l'écrit: La recherche avancé – Préface [Learning to Write: Advanced Research – Preface]. In: Marec-Breton, N., Besse, A-S, de La Haye, F., Bonneton-Botté N., Bonjour, E. (dir). *L'apprentissage de la langue écrite* [*Learning the written language*]. Rennes: Presse Universitaire de Rennes.

Gonçalves, B. A. G. & Capellini, S. M. A. (2010). Desempenho de escolares de 1ª série na bateria de identificação de erros de reversão e inversão na escrita: estudo preliminar [Performance of 1st grade students in the battery of identification of reversal errors and inversion in writing: preliminary study]. *Revista CEFAC,* 12 (6), 998-1008.

Guimarães, S. R. K., Paula, F. V. de. (2010). O papel da consciência morfossintática na aquisição e no aperfeiçoamento da leitura e da escrita [The role of morphosyntactic awareness in the acquisition and improvement of reading and writing]. *Educar em Revista*, 38:93-111. Editora UFPR

Jones, D. & Christensen, C. (1999). Relationship between automaticityin handwriting and students' ability to generate written text. *Journal of Educational Psychology,* 91(1), 44-9.

Kushki, A., Schwellnus, H., Iliyas F, Chau T. (2011). Changes in kinetics and kinematics of handwriting during a prolonged writing task in children with and without dysgraphia. *Research in Developmental Disabilities,* 32(3), 1058–1064. doi:10.1016/j.ridd.2011.01.026.

Lambert, E., Alamargot D., Larocque D. & Caporossi G. (2011). Dynamics of the spelling process during a copy task: effects of regularity and frequency. *Canadian Journal of Experimental Psychology*, 65(3), 141–150.doi: 10.1037/a0022538.

Lorenzini, M. V. (2003). *Uma escala para detectar a disgrafia baseada na escala de Ajuriaguerra.* (Dissertação de Mestrado) [*A scale for detecting dysgraphia based on the Ajuriaguerra scale.* (Masters dissertation)]. Universidade Federal de São Carlos. São Carlos – SP.

Maluf, M. R. (org.) (2003). *Metalinguagem e aquisição da escrita – Contribuições da pesquisa para a prática da alfabetização* [*Metalinguagem and acquisition of writing - Contributions of the research to the practice of literacy*]. São Paulo: Casa do Psicólogo.

Nicolson, R. & Fawcett, A. J. (2011). Dyslexia, dysgraphia, procedural learning and the cerebellum. *Cortex,* 47(1), 117-27.

Nobile, G. G. & Barrera, S. D. (2009). Análise de erros ortográficos em alunos do ensino público fundamental que apresentam dificuldades na escrita [Analysis of spelling errors in primary public school students who present difficulties in writing]. *Psicologia em revista,* 15(2), 36-55.

Okuda, P. M. M., Lourencetti, M. D., Santos, L. C. A., Padula, N. A. M. R. & Capellini, S. A. (2011). Coordenação motora fina de escolares com disgrafia e transtorno do déficit de atenção e hiperatividade [Fine motor coordination of schoolchildren with dysgraphia and attention deficit hyperactivity disorder]. *Revista CEFAC*, 13(5), 876-85.

Oliveira, R. M. S. G. (2000). *Aplicação da escala de disgrafia em crianças com e sem dificuldade na escrita* – (Dissertação de Mestrado) [*Application of dysgraphia scale in children with and without writing difficulties* - (Master's Dissertation)]. Universidade de Marília. Marília – SP.

Rotta, N. T., Ohweiler, L. & Riesgo, R. S. (2015). *Transtornos da aprendizagem: abordagem neurobiológica e multidisciplinary*

[*Learning Disorders: A Neurobiological and Multidisciplinary Approach*]. Porto Alegre: Artmed Editora. 512 páginas.

Rosenblum, S., Aloni, T. & Josman, N. (2010) Relationship between handwriting performance and organizational abilities among children with and without dysgraphia. A preliminary study. *Research in Developmental Disabilities*, 31(2), 502-9.

Reisman, J. E. (1993). Development and reliability of the research version of the Minnesota Handwriting Test. *Physical and Occupational Therapy in Pediatrics*, 13(2), 41–55.

Van Galen, G. P.; Meulenbroek, R. G. J.; Hylkema, H. (1986). On the simultaneous processing of words, letters and strokes in handwriting: evidences for a mixed linear and parallel mode. In: H. S. R Kao, G. P. Van Gallen, R. Roosain, (Orgs.). *Graphonomics: contemporary research in handwriting*. Amsterdam: Elsevier Science Publishers B. V. Chapter 1: 5-20.

Veloso, J. (2003). *Da influência do conhecimento ortográfico sobre o conhecimento fonológico: estudo longitudinal de um grupo de crianças falantes nativas do português europeu.* (Tese de Doutorado) [*From the influence of orthographic knowledge on phonological knowledge: longitudinal study of a group of native Portuguese speaking children.* (Doctoral thesis)]. Porto-Pt FLUP. http://hdl.handle.net/10216/18030.

Zesiger, P., Deonna, T. & Mayor C. (2000). L'acquisition de l'écriture [The acquisition of writing]. *Enfance,* 53(3), 295-304.

Zorzi, J. L. & Ciasca, S. M. A. (2008). Caracterização dos erros ortográficos em crianças com transtorno de aprendizagem [Characterization of orthographic errors in children with learning disorders]. *Revista CEFAC,* 10(3), 321-31.

In: Handwriting and Dysgrafia
Editors: M. Herrera Cardoso et al.
ISBN: 978-1-53613-805-4

Chapter 8

THE SPEED AND LEGIBILITY OF HANDWRITING IN DYSLEXIC STUDENTS

Monique Herrera Cardoso[1,*], Natália Lemes dos Santos[2,†] and Simone Aparecida Capellini[3,#]

[1]Education Program,
São Paulo State University "Júlio de Mesquita Filho" (UNESP),
Marília, São Paulo, Brazil
[2]Speech and Hearing Sciences School,
São Paulo State University "Júlio de Mesquita Filho" (UNESP),
Marília, São Paulo, Brazil
[3]Department of Speech and Hearing Sciences,
São Paulo State University "Júlio de Mesquita Filho" (UNESP),
Marília, São Paulo, Brazil

* Graduate Student; Corresponding Author: moniquehc@gmail.com
† Undergraduate; Corresponding Author: nlemess@gmail.com
# Full-Professor; Corresponding Author: sacap@uol.com.br

ABSTRACT

This chapter aims to compare the speed and legibility of handwriting of dyslexic students with the ones with good academic performance. Sixty-four students participated in the study; 07 dyslexic students of both genders, aged from 9 to 13 years and 1 month, composed group I (GI); and 57 students with good academic performance, of both genders, aged from 9 to 13 years and 1 month composed group II (GII). For the accomplishment of the study, the translated and adapted version of DASH was applied to Brazilian Portuguese, which consists of five tasks: Copy Best, Alphabet Writing, Copy fast of a sentence, Graphic speed and Free thematic writing. For the calculation of the writing speed, legible and illegible words per minute (LWPM/IWPM) were considered in the tasks Copy best, Copy fast of a sentence and Free thematic writing, the legible or illegible letters per minute (LLPM/ILPM) in the Alphabet Writing task, and the amount of "X" marked correctly in one minute in the Graphic speed task. It was possible to observe that GI presented inferior performance in LWPM and LLPM and superior performance in IWPM and ILPM, when compared to GII. In addition, GI still performed poorly on the Graphic speed task, when compared to GII students. Thus, it can be concluded that the performance in speed and legibility of writing of Brazilian dyslexics is inferior to students with good academic performance, and delay is observed in the percepto-viso-motor skills of dyslexics. Further studies are needed to investigate the correlation of calligraphy and motor skills, visual perceptive, attentional, memory and access to language codes, in order to better understand how these underlying factors may interfere and reflect on students' handwriting with dyslexia, in order to assist in the differential diagnosis and provide directions for health and education professionals, regarding interventions with calligraphic problems.

Keywords: assessment, dyslexia, handwriting

INTRODUCTION

Handwriting is considered a functional task used for communication and recoding of thoughts and experiences (Ziviani & Wallen, 2006). It is not an isolated motor act, but it is a complex skill which requires formal instruction since the early school years (Bosga-Stork, Bosga, &

Meulenbroek, 2015). To be properly developed, continuous interactions between the perceptual-motor processes and the cognitive processes are required (Graham, Berninger, Weintraub, & Schafer, 1998). The first one consists of visual perception, fine motor coordination and visual-motor integration; while the latter can be divided into more general processes, such as cognitive planning, work memory processes and more specific linguistic processes, such as phonological and orthographic coding (Simons & Probst, 2014).

A student needs to learn how to integrate all these skills (Lam, Au, Leung, & Li-Tsang, 2011), since handwriting is a continuous adaptive process of the perceptual-motor skills and attention abilities for language goals (Bosga -Stork et al., 2015). According to the literature (Longcamp et al., 2008), when handwriting is compared to the activity of typing the letters, favors letter recognition during reading, and also results into better spelling. When a student presents proficient writing, the execution of fast movements with the minimum of conscious effort, are expected (Tucha, Tucha, & Lange, 2008), that is, giving little or no attention to the process (Weigelt-Marom & Weintraub, 2018). Therefore, legibility means quality of letter formation, alignment and spacing of letters and words, and letter scaling (Feder, Majnemer, Bournonnais, Blayney, & Morin, 2001), and appropriate writing speed/letter production rate are fundamental (Kushki, Schwellnus, Faizah, & Chou, 2011) are fundamental (Amundson, 1995).

Difficulties concerning handwriting competence, throughout the school period, may cause long lasting negative effects on the students' academic success and upon self-esteem (Feder & Majnemer, 2007), making them avoid activities related to writing. This attitude is considered, in the view of parents and teachers, as an opposing behavior which generates conflicts at home and school (Racine, Majnemer, Shevell, & Snider, 2008). The prevalence of difficulties regarding handwriting is estimated between 10 and 30% (Feder and Majnemer, 2007; Kushki et al., 2011; Medwell & Wray, 2007), being manifested as illegible writing, slow writing speed, report of pain or discomfort during the activity, without any intellectual or somatic pathology (Overveld et al., 2011).

Although calligraphic difficulties are usual manifestations identified in students by teachers and professionals (Bosga-Stork et al., 2015), most of the times they are not considered as severe, and consequently, corrective actions are not performed (Lam et al., 2011). Students with non-proficient writing, present difficulties in the formation and sequencing of letters (Hoyles & Hoyles, 2010), higher pressures on the paper and greater variability in letter size (Brina, Niels, Overvelde, Levi, & Hulstijn, 2008). (Rosenblum, Aloni, & Josman, 2010), longer and unnecessary period of pencil/pen in the air (Rosenblum, Parush, & Weiss, 2003), more pauses during lettering (Chang & Yu, 2013) fewer characters written per minute, that is, they present slower writing speed than the proficient students (Rosenblum et al., 2003).

Currently, according to researches, different types of pathologies present difficulties in calligraphy (Cardoso & Capellini, 2016), such as autistic, attention deficit hyperactivity disorder (ADHD), developmental coordination disorder (DCD), among others. The study by Borella, Chicherio, Re, Sensini and Cornoldi (2011) states that students with dyslexia presented better performance in calligraphy compared to students with ADHD, however, when compared with typical students (Sumner, Connelly, & Barnett, 2013), dyslexics produce fewer letters/words per minute, characterizing a slow rate writing.

Difficulties in handwriting ability are not considered as a diagnostic criterion of any neurodevelopmental disorder yet (Lam et al., 2011), however, it is noted a prevalence of this difficulty in dyslexics when comparing with other cases of learning disorders (Martins et al., 2013). Although the World Health Organization (WHO, 1992) does not refer to difficulties of calligraphy for the definition of dyslexia, the Hong Kong Department of Education (HKSAR, 2002) has already included calligraphy deficiency as one of the main functional deficits in development (Ho, Chan, Lee, Tsang, & Luan, 2004).

Dyslexia is characterized as difficulties in decoding isolated words, usually reflecting inadequate phonological processing, unexpected in relation to age, and other cognitive and academic abilities, being able to interpret a heard text (Mousinho & Navas, 2016). According to Lyon,

Shaywitz and Shaywitz (2003), it is manifested by several linguistic difficulties, including reading alterations, problems with acquiring proficiency in writing and spelling.

According to DSM 5 (American Psychiatric Association, 2013) the term dyslexia refers to a pattern of learning difficulties characterized by problems with accuracy or fluency in recognizing words, impaired skills for decoding and spelling. A dyslexic student should present:

- Reading of words inaccurately or slowly, with some difficulties (e.g., reading isolated words aloud, incorrectly or slowly and hesitantly, often guesses words, has difficulty in spelling them).
- Difficulty in understanding the meaning of the text read (e.g., can read the text accurately, but does not understand the sequence, relationships, inferences, or deeper meanings of the text read).
- Difficulties in writing orthographically (e.g., add, omit, or replace vowels and consonants).
- Difficulties with written expressions (e.g., making multiple grammar or punctuation errors in sentences, employing inappropriate paragraph organization, written expressions of ideas without clarification).
- The affected academic skills are substantially and quantitatively below the expected for the student chronological age, causing significant interference in the academic or professional performance or daily activities, as confirmed by the standardized performance measures administered individually and by comprehensive clinical evaluation.
- Learning disabilities cannot be explained by intellectual impairments, uncorrected visual or auditory deficits, other neurological or mental disorders, psychosocial adversity, poor language proficiency for academic learning, or inadequate educational instruction.

- Difficulties in learning and using academic skills, as indicated by the presence of at least one of the following symptoms, which has persisted for at least 6 months, despite the provision of interventions targeting these difficulties.

Studies suggest that reading and writing may be indirectly interrelated (Chan, Ho, Tsang, Lee, & Chung, 2006; Tan, Spinks, Eden, Perfetti, & Siok, 2005), in which they may have underlying bonds with some cognitive abilities, such as orthographic perception and motor planning. However, researches with dyslexics have focused more deeply on reading problems (Berninger, Nielsen, Abbott, Wijsman, & Raskind, 2008) and associate writing difficulties with phonological deficits (Van Hoorn, Maathuis, Peters, & Hadders-Algra, 2010), neglecting calligraphy problems (Pagliarini et al., 2015).

Although it may be found in the international literature, studies (Borella et al., 2011; Sumner et al., 2013, Martins et al., 2013; Ho et al., 2004) investigating handwriting and writing speed of dyslexics (as reported previously), there are not publications regarding this theme in Brazil. This study intends to compare the speed and legibility of the handwriting of dyslexic students, with students with good academic performance, since it is believed that the Brazilian dyslexics performance will be lower than the typical students, as well as the researches of Lam et al. (2011) and Cheng-Lai, Li-Tsang, Chan and Lo (2013), who found out that speed and precision in calligraphy could differentiate Chinese children with dyslexia from typical children.

Studying performance variability, according to Nesselroade (1991), becomes important for health and education professionals to understand individual differences in the processes related to calligraphic writing learning, and, consequently, to define the best intervention program (Bosga-Stork et al., 2015) to minimize the difficulties of these students.

METHOD

Characterization of the Subjects

The students with diagnosis of dyslexia were selected for convenience, that is, they came from the Specialized Center for Rehabilitation of the Faculty of Philosophy and Sciences of São Paulo State University - CER II/FFC/UNESP- Marília- SP, who went through the multidisciplinary diagnostic process (including speech, neurological and neuropsychological assessment) in the first half of 2017, but were not submitted to any intervention session.

During this period, 7 dyslexic students of both genders, aged from 9 to 13 years and 1 month, agreed to participate in the study, which comprised group I (GI) of this study. Learning that dyslexia affects 5% to 17.5% of the school-age population (Lagae, 2008), a total of 57 students with good academic performance, of both genders, aged from 9 to 13 years and 1 month, were randomly selected (from a database of written samples), to comprise group II (GII), in order to pair with the GI dyslexics, so that 11% of the studied population presented dyslexia, that is, neither a minimum nor maximum for prevalence of dyslexia, but an intermediate prevalence for the diagnosis. Thus, this study included a total of 64 students.

As the research inclusion criteria, students should not present school records regarding auditory, visual, motor and/or intellectual deficiency, and could not present in their history any intervention (clinical and/or pedagogical) with focus on handwriting . According to resolution of the National Health Council CNS 196/96, prior to the beginning of the activities to be carried out, parents or guardians of the selected students signed the Informed Consent for authorization of the study, and 12-year-old students could sign the consent form. Failure to comply with at least one of the criteria described above, automatically excluded the student from the study sample.

Description of the Procedure Used

In order to perform this study, the instrument denominated Detailed Assessment of Speed of Handwriting - DASH (Barnett, Henderson, Scheib, & Schulz, 2007) was applied in the version translated and adapted for Brazilian Portuguese (Cardoso, Capellini, 2014), which we will denominated as DASH-PB, in this study.

The procedure consists of five tasks, which last approximately 30 minutes to be applied; four of them are writing tasks, and one of them consists on a measure of perceptual-motor competence. Data collection with the students was performed individually, in a single session, in which the five tasks proposed by DASH-PB were applied, as described below:

Task 1 – Copy best: copy a phrase (classified as a pangram) with best handwriting for two minutes;

Task 2 – Alphabet writing: write in lower case cursive letters the sequence of the alphabet, continuously, for one minute;

Task 3 – Copy fast of a sentence: Copy the same sentence from the first task, as fast as possible, but legibly, for two minutes;

Task 4 – Graphic speed: Make a series of "X" inside circles, for one minute;

Task 5 – Free thematic writing: Write a text about the theme "my life," for 10 minutes.

Data Analysis for Legibility

For tasks 1, 3 and 5, the researchers carried out the reading of each word written by the student only once; if they understood, the word should be classified as "legible," if they did not understand, they should not insist on re-reading, or should not "try" to understand by the context of the sentence, classifying it as" illegible." For task 2, the researchers only considered as "legible" the letters identified as lowercase cursive and alphabetically displayed; for uppercase, not written in alphabetical sequence, they were classified as "illegible." For task 4, since it was a perceptual-motor competence activity, it was not judged as to legibility, but rather the amount of "X" correctly and incorrectly marked inside the circles.

Writing Speed Calculation

The writing speed was calculated taking into account the amount of words (or letters in case of task 02) legible and illegible divided by minute, which will be presented in tasks 1, 3 and 5 as LWPM (legible words per minute) and IWPM (ilegible words per minute) and task 02 LLPM (legible letters per minute) and ILPM (ilegible letters per minute).

Data Analysis

To achieve the objective of this study, the data were analyzed statistically by SPSS software, version 20, through the ANOVA (Analysis of variance), which consists of a parametric test which compares the means by using variance. The use of a parametric statistical test is justified since the data are quantitative and continuous, however, a graphic analysis was previously done and found out that the data are approximate to a standard normal distribution and they present homocedasticity (constant variance). A significance level of 0.05 (5%) was defined, that is, all the confidence intervals presented 95% statistic al confidence.

RESULTS

Table 1 shows statistically significant differences in all comparisons between GI and GII, demonstrating that dyslexic students present inferior performance when compared to students with good academic performance in the five tasks proposed by the DASH-PB, characterizing lower writing speed and legibility.

Table 1. Comparison between dyslexic and typical schoolchildren in terms of writing speed (legible words)

		Groups	Media	Median	SD	IC	P-valor
Task 01	LWPM	Group I	7.79	8	3.57	2.64	0.023
		Group II	12.72	11.5	5.43	1.41	
Task 02	LLPM	Group I	13.43	13	4.04	2.99	0.026
		Group II	20.93	20	8.51	2.21	
Task 03	LWPM	Group I	7.64	7.5	2.14	1.58	<0.001
		Group II	16.39	16	5.47	1.42	
Task 04	Xs corrects	Group I	7.00	6	3.92	2.90	<0.001
		Group II	32.00	31	12.88	3.34	
Task 05	LWPM	Group I	6.30	5.8	2.93	2.17	0.058
		Group II	9.06	8.8	3.62	0.94	

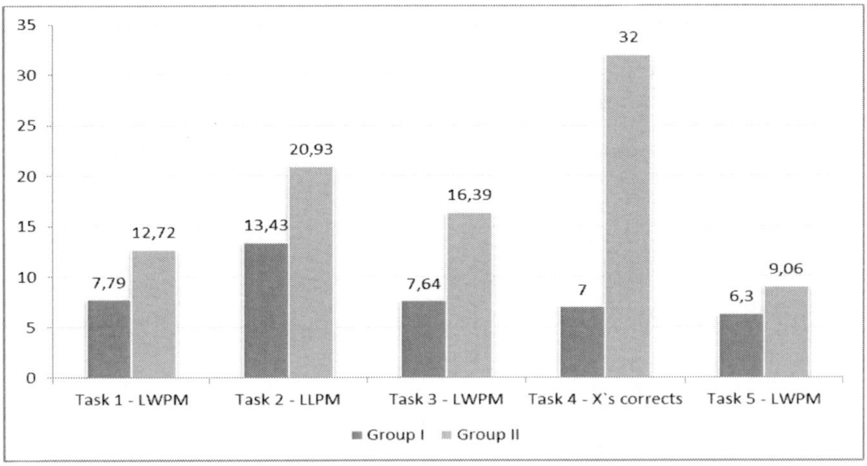

Graph 1. Comparison of averages in writing speed of legible words found for typical and dyslexic schoolchildren.

In Graph 1, this discrepancy between the two groups can be clearly observed, since GI presents lower average writing speed of legible words when compared with those with good academic performance. Finding of task 04 should be highlighted here, considering that dyslexic students presented a lower number of "X" correctly marked inside the circles, when compared to GII students.

Table 2. Comparison between dyslexic and typical schoolchildren when writing illegible words

		Groups	Media	Median	SD	IC	P-valor
Task 01	IWPM	Group I	1.64	1.5	1.77	1.31	<0.001
		Group II	0.04	0	0.26	0.07	
Task 02	ILPM	Group I	1.86	0	3.67	2.72	0.003
		Group II	0.28	0	0.56	0.15	
Task 03	IWPM	Group I	4.29	2.5	3.47	2.57	<0.001
		Group II	0.07	0	0.31	0.08	
Task 04	X`s incorrect	Group I	25.00	21	12.96	9.60	<0.001
		Group II	8.89	6	9.73	2.53	
Task 05	IWPM	Group I	2.71	1.4	2.45	1.82	<0.001
		Group II	0.04	0	0.08	0.02	

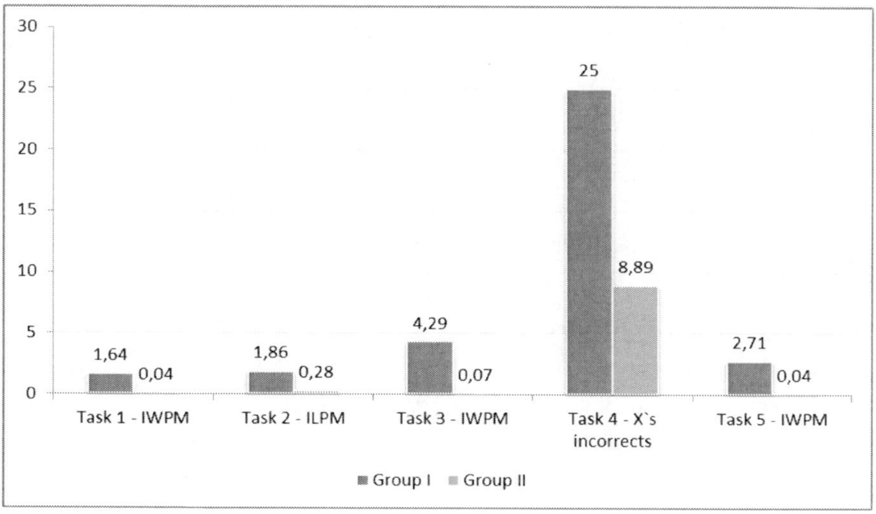

Graph 2. Comparison of the means of illegible words found for typical and dyslexic schoolchildren.

Table 2 shows a statistically significant difference between the groups in all DASH-PB applied tasks, characterizing that GI students present more illegible words than GII students.

In Graph 2, the discrepancy between the two groups can be observed once again, as GI presented higher averages of ilegible words, when compared to good academic performance students. It becomes worth highlighting the findings of task 04, since dyslexic students presented a higher amount of incorrectly marked "X" inside the circles, when compared to GII students.

DISCUSSION

As the objective of this study consists in comparing the speed and legibility of handwriting of dyslexic students with good academic performance students, it can be observed that the dyslexic present inferior performance than the ones with good academic performance, corroborating the literature (Cheng-Lai et al., 2013; Lam et al., 2011), as well as the chinese children, speed and precision in handwriting could differentiate Brazilian children with dyslexia, from typical children.

The recent study by Bosga-Stork et al., (2015) also states that dyslexic students can be identified through writing speed assessment, and this fact can be evidenced in this study, since in tasks concerning copying, alphabet writing and free thematic writing, the performance of dyslexics was lower, when compared to good academic performance students, thus, they presented less legible and more illegible words, in one minute.

The difference between students found in the tasks comcerning free thematic writing and alphabet writing, can be justified by the slow speed of dyslexics for accessing language codes, since there is a relationship between this ability and calligraphy (Peverly, Garner, & Vekaria, 2014). It can be observed, that in these tasks, the scholar should retrieve from memory the linguistic structure to be spelled out (words and/or letter) and the sequence of motor events to be performed for each letter; given the slowness in retrieving such information and difficulties at the rhythms of writing (Pagliarini et al., 2015), the speed and legibility of writing dyslexics may be altered.

As for copy tasks, differences between the students of both groups can be justified by fine motor difficulties, motor coordination deficit, balance, visual perception, visuospatial orientation, visual memory and viso-motor integration, which may be presented by dyslexics (Barnhardt, Borsting, Deland, Pham, & Vu, 2005; Capellini, Coppede, & Valle, 2010; Feder & Majnemer, 2007; Lam et al., 2011; Nicolson & Fawcett, 1990), since these impairments can affect legibility and variation in writing speed of these students.

Task 4, Graphic speed, presented the highest discrepancy between the groups performance, evidencing greater difficulty of dyslexics. As this task constitutes a perceptual-motor-visual assessment, it can be observed that these students presented alterations regarding this ability, and this fact was also evidenced in the study by McBride-Chang, Chung and Tong (2011), which identified that imprecision in writing of dyslexic students could be caused by developmental problems in visual-motor integration and attentive difficulties during the detailed formation of letters, thus affecting writing legibility.

According to Nicolson and Fawcett (1990; 2011), dysfunction in the cerebellum level of dyslexics could be considered as a hypothesis for justifying motor deficits and, therefore, could become an explanation for the co-occurrence between dysgraphia and dyslexia. However, it should be highlighted that students with dysgraphia are commonly identified, either by the school system or by health professionals, and thus should receive strategies for rehabilitation of handwriting, while dyslexic children do not undergo any kind of practical intervention concerning calligraphy, (Pagliarini et al., 2015), once the professionals' analyses are focused upon the other difficulties of these students, such as reading and spelling, leaving aside research and directed intervention towards handwriting of dyslexics.

Conclusion

Through this study, it was possible to confirm the hypothesis that the performance in speed and legibility of Brazilian dyslexic writing is inferior to students with good academic performance, and the perceptual-visual-motor skills of dyslexics are lower, when compared to the typical group.

However, new studies investigating the correlation of these abilities with calligraphy are necessary to obtain better understanding of how these underlying factors, such as motor skills, visual perception, attention, access memory to language codes, can interfere and reflect on the quality of handwriting.

Once further researches are concluded regarding the quality of handwriting of dyslexics, better diagnostic criteria will be available, besides favouring differential diagnosis concerning other neuro-developmental disorders, promoting guidelines for health professionals and education interventions towards the calligraphic problems of these students.

Acknowledgments

We are grateful to Capes (Coordination for Improvement of Higher Education Personnel) for the PhD scholarship granted to the first author.

References

American Psychiatric Association (2013). *Diagnostic and Statistical Manual of Mental Health Disorders*. 5th Edition. Arlington, VA: American Psychiatric Publishing.

Amundson, S. (1995). *Evaluation tool of children's handwriting*. Homer, AL: OT KIDS.

Barnett, A. L., Henderson, S. E., Scheib, B., & Schulz, J. (2007) *Detailed Assessment of Speed of Handwriting (DASH)*. United Kingdom: Person.

Barnhardt, C., Borsting, E., Deland, P., Pham, N., & Vu, T. (2005). Relationship between visual-motor integration and spatial organization of written language and math. *Optometry and Vision Science*, 82, 138–143.

Berninger, V. W., Nielsen, K. H., Abbott, R. D., Wijsman, E., & Raskind, W. (2008). Writing problems in developmental dyslexia: Under-recognized and undertreated. *Journal of School Psychology*, 46, 1–21.

Borella, E., Chicherio, C., Re, A. M., Sensini, V., & Cornoldi, C. (2011). Increased intraindividual variability is a marker of ADHD but also of dyslexia: A study on handwriting. *Brain and Cognition*,_77(1), 33-39. https://doi.org/10.1016/j.bandc.2011.06.005.

Bosga-Stork, I. M., Bosga, J., & Meulenbroek, R.G. J. (2015). Dysgraphic Handwriting Development and Inclusive Education: The Role of Interdisciplinary Counseling. *Open Journal of Social Sciences*, 3, 35-47. http://dx.doi.org/10.4236/jss.2015.38003.

Brina, C. D., Niels, R., Overvelde, A., Levi, G., & Hulstijn, W. (2008). Dynamic time warping: A new method in the study of poor handwriting. *Human Movement Science*, 27, 242–255.

Capellini, S., Coppede, A. C., & Valle, T. R. (2010). Fine motor function of school-aged children with dyslexia, learning disability and learning difficulties. *Pró-Fono Revista de Atualização Científica*, 23(3), 201–208.

Cardoso, M. H. (2014). *Adaptação Cultural do Detailed Assessment of Speed of Handwriting (DASH) para Escolares de Ensino Público*.118f. Dissertação (Mestrado em Fonoaudiologia) - Universidade Estadual Paulista/Faculdade de Filosofia e Ciências, Marília. Disponível em: <http://repositorio.unesp.br/bitstream/handle/11449/110549/000789304.pdf?sequence=1)>. Acesso em: 19 out. 2016. [*Cultural Adaptation of the Detailed Assessment of Speed of Handwriting (DASH) for Public School Teachers*.118f. Dissertation (Master degree in Speech Therapy).

Cardoso, M. H., & Capellini, S. A. (2016). Identificação e caracterização da disgrafia em escolares com dificuldades e transtornos de aprendizagem [Identification and characterization of dysgraphia in schoolchildren with learning difficulties and disorders]. *Distúrbios da Comunicação. 28*(1): 27-37. Disponível em: <https://revistas.pucsp.br/index.php/dic/article/view/23948/19268>. Acesso em: 23 jul 2017.

Cardoso, M. H., Henderson, S., & Capellini, S. A. (2014). Translation and cultural adaptation of Brazilian Detailed Assessment of Speed of Handwriting: conceptual and semantic equivalence. *Audiology Communication Research*, 19 (4), 321-326. Disponível em: <http://www.scielo.br/scielo.php?script=sci_arttext&pid=S2317-64312014000400321&lng=en&nrm=iso>. Acesso em: 24 ago 2017.

Chan, D. W., Ho, C. S. H., Tsang, S., Lee, S., & Chung, K. K. H. (2006). Exploring the reading-writing connection in Chinese children with dyslexia in Hong Kong. *Reading and Writing*, 19, 543–561.

Chang, S. H., & Yu, N. Y. (2013). Handwriting movement analyses comparing first and second graders with normal or dysgraphic characteristics. *Research in Developmental Disabilities*, 34(9), 2433–2441.

Cheng-Lai, A., Li-Tsang, C. W. P., Chan, A. H. L., & Lo, A. G. W. (2013). Writing to dictation and handwriting performance among Chinese children with dyslexia: Relationships with orthographic knowledge and perceptual-motor skills. *Research in Developmental Disabilities*, 34(10), 3372–3383. http://dx.doi.org/10.1016/j.ridd.2013.06.039.

Feder, K. P., Majnemer, A., Bournonnais, D., Blayney, M., & Morin, I. (2007). Handwriting performance on the ETCH-M in Grade One Regular Education Program. *Physical & Occupational Therapy in Pediatrics*, 2(2), 43-62.

Feder, K. P., & Majnemer, A. (2007). Handwriting development, competency, and intervention. *Developmental Medicine and Child Neurology*, 49, 312–317. Disponível em: gov.hk/UtilityManager/Publication/upload/sen_guide_e.pdf.

Graham, S., Berninger, V. W., Weintraub, N., & Schafer, W. (1998). Development of handwriting speed and legibility in Grades 1-9. *The Journal of Educational Research*, 92, 42-52.

Ho, C. S. H., Chan, D. W. O., Lee, S. H., Tsang, S. M., & Luan, V. H. (2004). Cognitive profiling and preliminary subtyping in Chinese developmental dyslexia. *Cognition*, 91, 43–75.

Hong Kong Education Department (2002). *Understanding and help students with special educational needs: A guide to teaching.* Disponível em: http://www.edb.gov.hk/UtilityManager/Publication/upload/sen_guide_e.pdf.

Hoyles, A., & Hoyles, M. (2010). Race and dyslexia. *Race Ethnicity*, 13, 209–231.

Kushki A., Schwellnus, H., Faizah, I., & Chou, T. (2011). Changes in kinetics and kinematics of handwriting during a prolongedwriting task in children with andwithout dysgraphia. *Research in Developmental Disabilities,* 32, 1058-1064.

Lagae, L. (2008). Learning disabilities: definitions, epidemiology, diagnosis, and intervention strategies. *Pediatric Clinics of North America*, 55(6), 1259-68.

Lam, S. S., Au, R. K., Leung, H. W., & Li-Tsang, C. W. P. (2011). Chinese handwriting performance of primary school children with dyslexia. *Research in Developmental Disabilities*, 32(5), 1745–1756. http://dx.doi.org/10.1016/j.ridd.2011.03.001.

Longcamp, M., Boucard, C., Gilhodes, J. C., Anton, J. L., Roth, M., Nazarian, B., & Velay, J. L. (2008) Learning through Hand- or Typewriting Influences Visual Recognition of New Graphic Shapes: Behavioral and Functional Imaging Evidence. *Journal of Cognitive Neuroscience*, 20 (5), 802-815. http://dx.doi.org/10.1162/jocn.2008.20504.

Lyon, G. R., Shaywitz, S. E., & Shaywitz, B. A. (2003). A definition of dyslexia. *Ann Dyslexia*, 53, 1-15.

Martins, M. R. I., Bastos, J. A., Cecato, A. T., Araujo, M. D. L. S., Magro, R. R., & Alaminos, V. (2013). Screening for motor dysgraphia in public schools. *Jornal de Pediatria (Versão em Português)*, *89*, 70-74. DOI: 10.1016/j.jped.2013.02.011.

McBride-Chang, C., Chung, K. K. H., & Tong, X. (2011). Copying skills in relation to word reading and writing in Chinese children with and without dyslexia. *Journal of Experimental Child Psychology*, 110, 422–433. http://dx.doi.org/10.1016/j.jecp.2011.04.014.

Medwell, J., & Wray, D. (2007). Handwriting: What do we know and what do we need to know? *Literacy*, 41, 10–15.

Mousinho, R., & Navas, A. L. (2016) Mudanças apontadas no DSM-5 em relação aos transtornos específicos de aprendizagem em leitura e escrita. *Revista debates em psiquiatria* [Changes pointed out in DSM-5 regarding specific learning disorders in reading and writing. *Journal debates in psychiatry*], 38-46. http://www.abp.org.br/rdp16/03/RDP_3_201604.pdf.

Nesselroade, J. R. (1991). The warp and woof of the developmental fabric. In R. Downs, L. Liben, & D. Palermo (Eds.), *Views of development, the environment, and aesthetics: The legacy of Joachim F. Wohlwill* (pp. 213–240). Hillsdale, NJ: Erlbaum.

Nicolson, R. I., & Fawcett, A. J. (1990). Automaticity: A new framework for dyslexia research? *Cognition*, 35, 159–182.

Nicolson, R. I., & Fawcett, A. J. (2011). Dyslexia, dysgraphia, procedural learning and the cerebellum. *Cortex*, 47(1), 117–127. http://dx.doi.org/10.1016/j.cortex.2009.08.016.

Overvelde, A., Bommel-Rutgers, I., Bosgra-Stork, I., Cauteren, Mv., Halfwerk, B., & Smits-Engelsman, B. C. (2011). Motorische schrijfproblemen bij kinderen. Nederlands Tijdschrift voor Fysiotherapie. *KNGF Evidence Statement* [Motor writing problems in children. *Dutch Journal for Physiotherapy*], 121, 1–65.

Pagliarini, E., Guasti, M. T., Toneatto C., Granocchio E., Riva F., Sarti D., Molteni B., & Stucchi N. (2015). Dyslexic children fail to comply with the rhythmic constraints of handwriting. *Human Movement Science*, 42, 161-182. https://doi.org/10.1016/j.humov.2015.04.012.

Peverly, S. T., Garner, J. K., & Vekaria, P. C. (2014). Both handwriting speed and selective attention are important to lecture note-taking. *Reading and Writing*, 27(1), 1–30. https://doi.org/10.1007/s11145-013-9431-x.

Racine, M. B., Majnemer, A., Shevell, M., & Snider, L. (2008). Handwriting performance in children with attention deficit hyperactive disorder (ADHD). *Journal of Child Neurology*, 23, 399–406.

Rosenblum, S., Aloni, T., & Josman, N. (2010). Relationships between handwriting performance and organizational abilities among children with and without dysgraphia: A preliminary study. *Research in Developmental Disabilities*, 31(2), 502–509.

Rosenblum, S., Parush, S., & Weiss, P. L. (2003). Computerized temporal handwriting characteristics of proficient and nonproficient handwriters. *The American Journal of Occupational Therapy*, 57(2), 129–138.

Simons, J., & Probst, M. (2014). Reliability of the Detailed Assessment of Speed of Handwriting on Flemish Children. *Pediatric Physical Therapy*, 26 (3), 318–324. doi: 10.1097/PEP.0000000000000050.

Sumner, E., Connelly, V., & Barnett, A. L. (2013). Children with dyslexia are slow writers because they pause more often and not because they are slow at handwriting execution. *Reading and Writing*, *26*(6), 991-1008. http://dx.doi.org/10.1007/s11145-012-9403-6.

Tan, L. H., Spinks, J. A., Eden, G. F., Perfetti, C. A., & Siok, W. T. (2005). Reading depends on writing, in Chinese. *Proceedings of the National Academy of Sciences of the United States of America*, 102, 8781–8785.

Tucha, O., Tucha, L., & Lange, K. W. (2008). Graphonomics, automaticity and handwriting assessment. *Literacy*, 42(3), 145–155.

Van Hoorn, J. F., Maathuis, C. G. B., Peters, L. H. J., & Hadders-Algra, M. (2010). Handwriting, visuomotor integration, and neurological condition at school age. *Developmental Medicine and Child Neurology*, 52, 941–947.

Weigelt-Marom, H., & Weintraub, N. (2018). Keyboarding versus handwriting speed of higher education students with and without learning disabilities: Does touch-typing assist in narrowing the gap?

Computers & Education, 117, 132-140. https://doi.org/10.1016/j.compedu.2017.10.008.

World Health Organization (1992). *The ICD-10 classification of mental and behavioural disorders:* Clinical descriptions and diagnostic guidelines. Geneva: World Health Organization.

Ziviani, J., & Wallen, M. (2006). The development of graphomotor skills. In A. Henderson, & C. Pehoski (eds), *Hand Function in the Child. Foundations for Remediation*. (2, pp. 217-238) ed. St Louis, MO: Mosby Elsevier.

In: Handwriting and Dysgrafia
Editors: M. Herrera Cardoso et al.
ISBN: 978-1-53613-805-4

Chapter 9

THE RELATIONSHIP BETWEEN VISO-MOTOR SKILLS AND HANDWRITING IN STUDENTS WITH DYSLEXIA

***Simone Aparecida Capellini*[1,*], *Flávia Santana Serrão*[2], *Noemi Del Bianco*[3,†], *Giseli Donadon Germano*[4] and *Catia Giaconi*[5]**

[1]Department of Speech and Hearing Sciences,
São Paulo State University "Júlio de Mesquita Filho" (UNESP),
Marília, São Paulo, Brazil
[2]Investigation Learning Disabilities Laboratory,
Department of Speech and Hearing Sciences,
São Paulo State University "Júlio de Mesquita Filho" (UNESP),
Marília, São Paulo, Brazil
[3]Human Sciences, Education,
University of Macerata, Macerata, Italy
[4]Department of Special Education,
São Paulo State University "Júlio de Mesquita Filho" (UNESP),
Marília, São Paulo, Brazil

---

* Full Professor; Corresponding Author: sacap@uol.com.br
† PhD in Human Sciences, Education

[5]Didactic and Special Pedagogy, Department of Education, Cultural Heritage and Tourism, University of Macerata, Macerata, Italy

ABSTRACT

Aim: To relate the viso-motor skills and handwriting of students with dyslexia.

Methods: Twenty-two students with multidisciplinary diagnosis of dyslexia, aged from 8 years and 3 months to 13 years and 4 months, of both genders, from third to fifth grade of elementary school participated in this study. The students were submitted to the following procedures: Visual Perception Development Test III - DTVP III and Dysgraphia Scale.

Results: The results indicated that most students with dyslexia were classified as dysgraphics. Therefore, from the analysis of the Visual Perception Development Test (DTVP-III) it was possible to observe that there was an impact of the variables related to the visomotor and fine motor skills.

Conclusion: Nevertheless, the findings of this study indicate that dyslexic students presented difficulties in visomotor skills, thus impairing hand writing. Thus, most of these students presented compatible performance for disgraphic writing.

Keywords: handwriting, dyslexia, viso-motor perception

INTRODUCTION

Dyslexia refers to a specific learning disorder impairing reading, which occurrs at the beginning of literacy, affecting reading acquisition, handwriting, and spelling (Reid, 2013).

In relation to handwriting, studies indicated that students with dyslexia may present dysgraphia, which is characterized by difficulties in the acquisition of writing skills, with writing performance lower than expected to the class level of children (Döhla & Heim, 2016; McCloskey & Rapp, 2017). The prevalence of dysgraphia was described as 7 to 15% of students, thus boys are more affected than girls, proportion between 2-3

(Hawke, Olson, Willcut, Wadsworth, & DeFries, 2009; Katusic, Colligan, Weaver, & Barbaresi, 2009).

As described by Crawford and Dewey (2008), the necessity of investigating and acknowledging the perceptual-motor performance of students with dyslexia lies in the fact that many of the alterations in writing, identified as spelling mistakes, may actually be masking calligraphic errors, such as: badly traced letter which triggers unintelligible writing.

Thus, Tseng and Chow (2000) reported that students with dyslexia may present difficulties regarding letter tracing and speed, which are related to impairments in visual perception or deficient underlying cognitive abilities.

Goulandris and Snowling (1991), have also suggested that deficits in the visual domain may lead to dysgraphia. The authors reported that impairments in visual memory may cause difficulties for retention of information necessary for the construction of long-term memory orthographic representations.

In regard to the development of handwriting, the required motor control is quite demanding, and the process of learning letters occurs in a slow and variable way, being automated around 10-11 years. Thus, when automated, the student can devote himself to other types of learning, such as sentence construction and writing (Pontart et al., 2013). Kandel and Perret (2015) report that with automation, there is also a greater interaction between orthographic (central process) and motor processing levels (peripheral processes) (McCloskey & Rapp, 2017).

Thus, one of the important aspects related to handwriting irefers to viso-motor integration, which can be defined as an integration between visual perception and motor skills, that is, it involves the ability to identify and process visual information related to motor function, such as eye-hand coordination (Lahav, Apter, & Ratzonl, 2013; Pereira, Araújo, & Braccialli, 2011). Thus, the student who does not develop this ability may present difficulties in writing, concerning its quality (Feder & Majnemer, 2007).

However, other subjacent processes occur, as the cognitive functions: voluntary attention, motor planning, scheduling and verification of motor effectiveness, if necessary for reprogramming. Thus, visual and tactile-kinesthetic feedbacks take active part in this writing production process (Germano, Pinheiro, Okuda, & Capellini, 2013).

Thus, for handwriting production, the students' needs visual perception skills, to construct internal representations of visual information, which provide characteristics such as: shape, size, position in space and distance from letters. It also becomes necessary to improve motor and sensory-motor coordination functions, from which the student receives tactile-kinesthetic information, maintaining adequate gripping and pressure movements during writing, as well as proper sequencing of manual movements (Andrade et al., 2012; Fusco, Okuda, & Capellini 2011; Okuda, Lourencetti, Santos, Padula, & Capellini 2011; Vinter & Chartrel, 2010).

Finally, the student needs viso-motor integration skills, which allows the execution of copy or transposition of texts, production of cursive letters, reproduction of letters and numbers isolated and in sequences (Brown & Rodger, 2008; Brown, Unsworth & Lyons, 2009).

Thus, the final steps in the writing process involve the conversion of motor-graphic planning into specific motor-action programs and the employment of this planning by the motor system to perform the appropriate writing movements. During the writing process, the visual feedback plays an important role, not only to ensure proper orientation and spacing of letters and words throughout the page, but also for monitoring and controlling letter forms, individually (McCloskey & Rapp, 2017).

According to the above, the objective of this chapter was to relate viso-motor skills and handwriting in students with dyslexia.

MATERIAL AND METHOD

This study was approved by the Research Ethics Committee of the Faculty of Philosophy and Sciences of São Paulo State University "Júlio de

Mesquita Filho" (UNESP) Marília, São Paulo, Brazil), number CAAE 40514615.8.0000.5406.

Twenty-two students with multidisciplinary diagnosis of dyslexia, aged from 8 years and 3 months to 13 years and 4 months; 55% females and 45% males, participated in this study. From these students, 37% attended the third grade of Elementary School, 37% the fourth grade, and 26% the fifth grade.

The students were diagnosed by a multidisciplinary team from the Investigation Learning Disabilities Laboratory, Department of Speech and Hearing Sciences, São Paulo State University "Júlio de Mesquita Filho" (UNESP), Marília, São Paulo, Brazil and were not submitted to intervention procedures prior to the beginning of this research.

The students were submitted individually to the following procedures:

- *Visual Perception Developmental Test III - DTVP III* (Hammill, Pearson, & Voress, 2014): this protocol is composed of subtests: eye-hand coordination (EH), Copy (CO), Figure - Ground (FG), Visual Closure (VC) and Form Constancy (FC). The score is performed in standard score and composed score, being classified from total score and its conversion by using tables, and composed score. The composed score allows classification in relation to general visual perception (IMV, composed by subtests: copy, eye-hand coordination, figure-ground, visual closure, and form constancy), reduced motor perception (MRVP, composed by subtests: figure-ground, visual closure and form constancy) and viso-motor integration (GVP, composed by subtests: copy and eye-hand coordination). The students were classified in relation to the composed scores, such as: "very poor" (1), "poor" (2), "below average" (3), "average" (4), "above average", "Superior" (6) and "very superior" (7).
- *Dysgraphia Scale* (Lorenzini, 1993): Writing analysis was performed through the application of the Dysgraphia Scale (Lorenzini, 1993), composed of 10 evaluation items to be written as dictation (floating lines, ascending/descending lines, irregular

space between words, retouched letters, curvatures at angles of the arches of M, N, U, V, junction points, collisions and adhesions, sudden movements, irregular dimensions and bad forms). The punctuation criterion employed to analyze the students' writing performance of this study is proposed by (Lorenzini, 1993), and the overall grade (ou score) for each writing ranged from zero to seventeen points; thus, every subject who obtained score equal or superior to eight and a half points - equivalent to 50% of the total score, was considered as dysgraphic.

Data collection was performed into 4 sessions, each one lasting 40 minutes, during one month.

Statistical Analysis

The results were analyzed statistically, through the employment of the *Spearman Correlation Analysis Test*. The results were statistically analyzed at the significance level of 5% (0.050), indicated with asterisks on the tables referring to the results. The degree of relationship was analyzed according to the criteria of direction and strength. The positive direction happens when there is an indication of a linear relationship, that is, when one of the variables increases, the other one also increases. In other words, the variables are directly proportional. Yet, the negative direction indicates that when there is an increase in one variable, there is a decrease in the other, that is, the variables are indirectly proportional. As for strength, when it is closer to 1, the stronger the linear association between the two variables and the sign of the correlation coefficient (ie, positive or negative) defines the direction of the relation. The absolute value indicates correlation strength (Zou, Tunacall, & Silverman, 2003).

Table 1 shows the mean and standard deviation of the Visual Perception Performance Test (DTVP-III) and the Dysgraphia Scale. Regarding the dysgraphia scale, it is worth noting that 72.7% of the dyslexics in this study were classified as dysgraphic.

Table 2 presents the Spearman correlation analysis between the Visual Perception Performance Test (DTVP-III) and the Dysgraphia Scale.

Table 1. Mean and standard deviation of the Visual Perception Performance Test (DTVP-III) and the Dysgraphia Scale

	Variables	Mean	Standard Deviation
Visual Perception Developmental Test III - DTVP III	EH	155.91	25.230
	CO	29.27	7.376
	FG	36.55	14.060
	VC	12.27	3.480
	FC	30.09	7.922
	CL_EH	2.82	1.736
	CL_CO	4.05	1.362
	CL_FG	2.82	1.368
	CL_VC	2.95	1.090
	CL_FC	3.23	0.922
	CL_VMI	3.14	1.670
	CL_MRVP	2.45	1.143
	CL_GVP	2.86	1.207
Dysgrap hia Scale	LF	1.14	0.834
	LDA	0.727	0.2979
	EI	0.17	0.389
	LR	1.32	0.839
	CAA	0.364	0.4676
	PJ	0.82	0.853
	CA	1.295	1.4853
	MB	1.68	0.716
	ID	1.55	0.739
	MF	0.78	0.428
	T	9.977	3.5135
	CL_D	0.73	0.456

Legend: LF: Floating lines, LD/A: Descending and/or ascending lines, EI: Irregular Spaces between words, LR: Rectangled Letters, CA/A: Curvatures and Angulations of M, N, V and U arcades, PJ : Junction points, CA: collision and adhesions, MB: Hard Movements, ID: dimension irregularity, MF: More Forms. CL: Classification; D: Dysgraphia; EH: hand-eye coordination, CO: copy; FG: Figure - Ground, VC: Visual Closure (VC), FC: Form Constancy; VMI: general visual perception; MRVP: reduced motor perception; GVP: general visual perception.

Table 2. Spearman correlation analysis between the Visual Perception Performance Test (DTVP-III) and the Dysgraphia Scale

		EH	CO	FG	VC	FC	CL_EH	CL_CO	CL_FG	CL_VC	CL_FC	CL_VMI	CL_MRVP	CL_GVP
LF	ρ	-0.107	0.012	-0.265	0.127	-0.156	-0.001	-0.167	-0.330	0.195	-0.160	-0.107	-0.161	-0.106
	p value	0.634	0.959	0.234	0.573	0.489	0.996	0.458	0.133	0.384	0.477	0.634	0.475	0.638
LDA	ρ	-0.069	-0.212	-0.011	-0.166	0.103	-0.022	0.102	0.130	0.051	0.050	0.008	0.286	0.062
	p value	0.761	0.344	0.961	0.461	0.649	0.923	0.653	0.565	0.821	0.824	0.970	0.196	0.784
EI	ρ	0.194	0.648	0.519	0.652	0.585	0.407	0.070	0.210	0.000	0.102	0.422	0.103	0.000
	p value	0.545	**0.023***	0.084	**0.021***	**0.046***	0.189	0.830	0.513	1.000	0.754	0.172	0.750	1.000
LR	ρ	-0.245	-0.294	-0.174	-0.031	-0.343	-0.284	-0.012	0.068	0.280	0.002	-0.164	0.103	0.239
	p value	0.271	0.184	0.439	0.892	0.118	0.199	0.959	0.764	0.207	0.992	0.467	0.648	0.284
CAA	ρ	0.297	0.378	0.608	0.450	0.687	0.245	0.325	0.460	0.206	0.359	0.240	0.430	0.394
	p value	0.179	0.083	**0.003***	**0.036***	**0.000***	0.271	0.140	**0.031***	0.358	0.100	0.283	**0.046***	0.069
PJ	ρ	-0.239	-0.364	-0.336	-0.385	-0.448	-0.248	-0.322	-0.264	-0.020	-0.064	-0.136	-0.275	-0.111
	p value	0.284	0.096	0.126	0.077	**0.036***	0.267	0.144	0.234	0.928	0.777	0.545	0.215	0.624
CA	ρ	0.026	0.244	0.571	0.388	0.521	-0.042	0.245	0.478	0.150	0.219	0.042	0.343	0.266
	p value	0.908	0.274	**0.006***	0.074	**0.013**	0.853	0.271	**0.024***	0.506	0.328	0.852	0.118	0.232
MB	ρ	-0.173	-0.058	0.128	0.340	-0.072	-0.084	-0.022	0.054	0.401	-0.095	0.072	0.245	0.235
	p value	0.442	0.799	0.569	0.121	0.751	0.709	0.923	0.810	0.065	0.674	0.749	0.271	0.292
ID	ρ	0.115	0.057	-0.085	-0.090	0.138	0.115	-0.250	-0.211	-0.111	-0.056	-0.032	-0.207	-0.121
	p value	0.609	0.802	0.707	0.690	0.540	0.610	0.262	0.347	0.623	0.803	0.886	0.356	0.591
MF	ρ	0.335	-0.168	0.129	0.297	0.271	0.345	-0.128	0.027	0.246	0.243	0.082	0.267	0.202
	p value	0.174	0.506	0.610	0.231	0.276	0.161	0.614	0.915	0.325	0.330	0.746	0.285	0.422
T	P	-0.036	0.121	0.193	0.300	0.230	-0.025	0.087	0.150	0.316	0.138	0.036	0.251	0.264
	p value	0.874	0.591	0.389	0.176	0.303	0.913	0.702	0.506	0.151	0.539	0.874	0.260	0.236
CL_D	*P*	-0.169	-0.113	0.000	0.331	-0.137	-0.042	-0.081	-0.077	0.431	-0.102	0.043	0.158	0.188
	p value	0.452	0.617	1.000	0.132	0.543	0.854	0.719	0.733	**0.045***	0.651	0.851	0.483	0.403

Legend: LF: Floating lines, LD/A: Descending and/or ascending lines, EI: Irregular Spaces between words, LR: Rectangled Letters, CA/A: Curvatures and Angulations of M, N, V and U arcades, PJ : Junction points, CA: collision and adhesions, MB: Hard Movements, ID: dimension irregularity, MF: More Forms. CL: Classification; D: Dysgraphia; EH: hand-eye coordination, CO: copy; FG: Figure - Ground, VC: Visual Closure (VC), FC: Form Constancy; VMI: general visual perception; MRVP: reduced motor perception; GVP: general visual perception.

Table 2 shows a moderate positive relation between irregular space (EI), of the Dysgraphia Scale and Copy (CO), Visual Closure (VC) and Form Constancy (FC) of DTVP-III, indicating that the better the visual closure skill ability and consistency of writing words without irregular space between them; there was a moderate positive relation between Curvature and Angulations of the arches of M, N, V and U (CA/A) of the Dysgraphia Scale and Figure-Ground (FG), Visual Closure (VC), Form Constancy (FC), classification figure-ground (FG) and reduced motor perception (MRVP) indicating that the better the perception of reduced motricity,, the better the curvature and angulation of the letters M, N, V and U; there was a moderate positive relation between DTVP - III collision and adhesion (AC) of the Scale of dysgraphy and Figure-Ground (FG), Form Constancy (FC) and Figure-Ground classification (FG) of DTVP-III indicating that the better the figure-ground skill, the better the form constancy, better the writing quality, without adherent letters or collision; of the students. There was a moderate positive correlation between dysgraphia classification of the dysgraphia scale and the figure-ground classification (FG of DTVP-III, indicating that the better the figure-ground, the better the quality of the students' writing. There was moderate negative correlation between junction points (PJ) Scale of Dysgraphia and Form Constancy (FC) of DTVP-III indicating that the better the form constancy, there are fewer junction points in writing.

Discussion

Motor visual integration (VMI), as an ability to use input information from the percepto-visual system to coordinate fine motor skills, requires the use of smaller muscles of wrist and hand, including dexterity, precision, coordination, and manual control (Schneck, 2010), and these associations are present in daily activities, such as: calligraphy and drawing, catching a ball, dressing, eating, and so on. (Tomchek & Schneck, 2006; Doney et al., 2016).

When assessed separately, VMI integration is directly related to grafomotricity (Beery & Beery, 2010; Kulp, 1999; Milner & Goodale, 2006) indicating that the presence of alterations in this integrative ability may result into problems underlying visual perception or fine motor skills.

Based on the findings of this study, students with dyslexia presented difficulties related to visual abilities (Visual Closure, Form Constancy, and Figure - Ground when compared to visual-motor integration skills (Copy).

The results indicated a positive and moderate relationship between the visual abilities, such as: Figure-Background, Visual Closure, and Form Constancy of the Visual Perception and Irregular Space (EI) tests, Curvatures and Angulations of the M, N, V and U arches, collision and adherence of the Scale of Dysgraphia, suggesting that the difficulty in the domain of these visual abilities may impair the execution of some manual writing aspects, such as: motor planning of straight lines and curvatures and the space between letters and words.

Regarding the visual abilities described above, Martin (2006), mentioned that they are related to learning how to write, since they enable the student to discriminate between letter detailing and general word configuration (a - o; f - t; n - u). Cardoso & Capellini (2012), reported that visual skills as figure-ground, visual closure and form constancy are directly related to handwriting, since the graphomotor action depends on the detail recognition, simultaneous processing, visuospatial organization, spatial relation between the figures of integration of the parts of a whole, giving meanings to the forms of the letters, and consequently, affecting the graphomotor performance for the production of these letters.

Thus, the students of this study presented difficulties concerning the perception of letter details, as verified in the score of Curvatures and Angulations of the M, N, V and U (CA/A) arches of the Dysgraphia Scale. For this item of the Dysgraphia Scale, the student should perform straight line (straight stems) and curvature (rounded) movements in the medial region of the letter, thus making an angulation, which specifically characterizes each of these letters, according to described by Lorenzini (1993).

The students of this study also presented difficulties in relation to the item collision and adhesions. For accomplishment this item, the student should avoid flattening one letter over another (Lorenzini, 1993). Thus, he should plan the layout of each letter of the word, adjusting the form and distance between them, so that this viso-spatial information must be constantly verified through visual feedback. Handwriting requires information about the form of the letter that the student retains in his memory, and the movements are adjusted from the visual feedback.

The relation between visual skills and dysgraphia was described by Martin (2006), since, to form a visual image of letters and words during writing production, the student should perceive the position of letters in space and recognize visual cues and/or fragments that will favor words tracing, giving an appearance of final product (writing). Tseng and Chow (2000) also reported that difficulties in tracing letters can be related to visual perception impairments, which influence motor action planning.

There was also, in this study, a negative and moderate relation between the visual ability of Form Constancy and the Dysgraphia Scale Junction Point, suggesting that the perception that letters can have the same tracing, regardless of size, they should remain together to form a word, fluent, without bonding one letter to another, within the same word, making writing unintelligible.

Goulandris and Snowling (1991) stated that, for the formation of visual memory of letters, the student should perceive repeated details (straight lines, curvatures) and they will be associated to a graphomotor representation. From this perception, handwriting will be a visual memory product (core processes), which contains orthographic representations and motor planning in long-term memory. Thus, writing observed on paper constitutes a final product, resulting from so many other central and peripheral processes (Kandel & Perret, 2015; McCloskey & Rapp, 2017), which in this study was verified through the Scale of Dysgraphia.

In relation to the students of this study, it was observed that most of the dyslexics presented dysgraphic writing. Gomes (2009) and Fusco (2013), reported that students with dyslexia may present visual information processing impairments which could justify the presence of dysgraphia.

Bellocchi et al., (2017), reported that dyslexics demonstrated impairments in Visual Closure, Form Constancy, and Figure–Ground, when compared to students with good academic performance.

Conclusion

Based on the findings of this study, it can be concluded that there was a relationship between viso-motor skills and writing quality, indicating that the dysgraphic writing of students with dyslexia is marked by the relationship between irregular space (EI), of the Scale of Dysgraphy and Copy, Visual Closure (VC) and Form Constancy (FC) of the DTVP-III relationship between the curvatures and angulations of M, N, V and U (CA/A) of the Scale of Dysgraphia and Figure-Ground (FG) Visual Closure (VC), Form Constancy (FC), Figure - Ground (FG) classification and reduced motor perception (MRVP), relationship between collision and adhesion (CA) of the Scale of Dysgraphia and Figure - Ground (FG) Form Constancy (FC) and classification Figure-Ground, relation between the classification of the Scale of Dysgraphia and Classification Figure-Ground-FG of DTVP-III; relation between Junction Points (PJ) of the Dysgraphia Scale and Form Constancy of DTVP –III.

References

Andrade, S. M., Dias, M. M. C. D. B., Oliveira, E. A. D., Locks Neto, F., Nogueira, R. M. T. B. L., & Santos, N. A. D. (2012). Construction and psychometric evidences of a visual perception scale. *Psicologia: Reflexão e Crítica*, 25(1), 21-29. DOI: 10.1590/S0102-7972201200 0100004.

Beery, K. E., & Beery, N. A. (2010). Beery VMI.: The Beery-Buktenica Developmental Test of Visual-motor Integration with Supplemental Developmental Tests of Visual Perception and Motor Coordination:

And, Stepping Stones Age Norms from Birth to Age Six. *Administration, Scoring, and Teaching Manual*. PsychCorp.

Bellocchi, S., Muneaux, M., Huau, A., Lévêque, Y., Jover, M., & Ducrot, S. (2017). Exploring the Link between Visual Perception, Visual–Motor Integration, and Reading in Normal Developing and Impaired Children using DTVP- 2. *Dyslexia*, 23(3), 296-315. DOI:10.1002/dys.1561.

Brown, T., & Rodger, S. (2008). Validity of the developmental test of visual-motor integration supplemental developmental test of visual perception. *Perceptual and motor skills*, 106(3), 659-678. DOI:10.2466/pms.106.3.659-678.

Brown, T., Unsworth, C., & Lyons, C. (2009). An evaluation of the construct validity of the Developmental Test of Visual- Motor Integration using the Rasch Measurement Model. *Australian occupational therapy journal*, *56*(6), 393-402. DOI: 10.1111/j.1440-1630.2009.00811.x.

Cardoso M. H., Capellini S. A. Ocorrência da disgrafia em escolares com dificuldades e transtornos de aprendizagem. [Occurrence of dysgraphia in schoolchildren with learning difficulties and disorders.] In: Capellini SA, Sampaio MN, Oliveira AM, orgs. *Tópicos em transtornos de aprendizagem II: ênfase na perspectiva interdisciplinar.* 1ª ed. São José dos Campos: Pulso Editorial; 2012. p. 21-34.

Crawford, S. G., & Dewey, D. (2008). Co-occurring disorders: a possible key to visual perceptual deficits in children with developmental coordination disorder? *Human movement science*, 27(1), 154-169. DOI:10.1016/j.humov.2007.09.002.

Döhla, D., & Heim, S. (2016). Developmental dyslexia and dysgraphia: What can we learn from the one about the other? *Frontiers in psychology*, 26 (6), 2045. DOI:10.3389/fpsyg.2015.02045.

Doney, R., Lucas, B. R., Watkins, R. E., Tsang, T. W., Sauer, K., Howat, P., ... & Elliott, E. J. (2016). Visual-motor integration, visual perception, and fine motor coordination in a population of children with high levels of Fetal Alcohol Spectrum Disorder. *Research in developmental disabilities*, *55*, 346-357 DOI: 10.1016j.ridd.2016. 05.009.

Feder K. P., Majnemer A. Handwriting development, competency, and intervention. *Dev Med Child Neurol*. 2007; 49(4):312-7. DOI: 10.1111/j.1469-8749.2007.00312.x.

Fusco, N., Okuda, P. M. M., & Capellini, S. A. (2011). Avaliação e intervenção com a habilidade visomotora em escolares com dislexia e distúrbio de aprendizagem [Evaluation and intervention with the visomotor ability in schoolchildren with dyslexia and learning disorder]. In S. A. Capellini, C. Silva, & F. H. Pinheiro (Org.). *Tópicos em transtornos de aprendizagem* [*Topics in learning disorders*]. (pp. 79-89). São José dos Campos: Pulso Editorial,

Fusco, N. (2013). *Elaboração de programa de intervenção com as habilidades percepto-viso-motoras em escolares com dislexia do desenvolvimento* (Dissertação de mestrado) [*Elaboration of an intervention program with perceptual-motor skills in schoolchildren with developmental dyslexia* (Master's Dissertation)]. Universidade Estadual Paulista (UNESP), Marília, SP.

Germano, G. D., Pinheiro, F. H., Okuda, P. M. M., & Capellini, S. A. (2013). Visual-motor perception in students with Attention Deficit with Hyperactivity Disorder. *CoDAS*, 25 (4), 337-341. DOI: 10.1590/ S2317-17822013000400007.

Gomes Z. G. Neurofisiologia da linguagem oral e escrita [Neurophysiology of oral and written language]. In: Zorzo J, Capellini, AS. *Dislexia do desenvolvimento e outros distúrbios de leitura-escrita.* [*Developmental dyslexia and other reading-writing disorders*]. São José dos Campos (SP): Pulso; 2009. p. 35-42.

Goulandris, N. K., & Snowling, M. (1991). Visual memory deficits: A plausible cause of developmental dyslexia? Evidence from a single case study. *Cognitive Neuropsychology*, 8(2), 127-154. DOI:10.1080/ 02643299108253369.

Hammill, D. D., Pearson, N. A., & Voress, J. K. (1993). *Developmental Test of Visual Perception: DTVP-2*. Austin, TX: Pro-ed.

Hawke, J. L., Olson, R. K., Willcut, E. G., Wadsworth, S. J., & DeFries, J. C. (2009). Gender ratios for reading difficulties. *Dyslexia*, 15(3), 239-242. DOI: 10.1002/dys.389.

Kandel, S., & Perret, C. (2015). How does the interaction between spelling and motor processes build up during writing acquisition? *Cognition,* 136, 325-336.

Katusic, S. K., Colligan, R. C., Weaver, A. L., & Barbaresi, W. J. (2009). The forgotten learning disability: epidemiology of written-language disorder in a population-based birth cohort (1976–1982), Rochester, Minnesota. *Pediatrics,* 123(5), 1306-1313. DOI: 1 0.1016/j.cognition. 2014.11.014.

Kulp, M. T. (1999). Relationship between visual motor integration skill and academic performance in kindergarten through third grade. *Optometry and vision science,* 76(3), 159-163.

Lahav, O., Apter, A., & Ratzon, N. Z. (2013). Psychological adjustment and levels of self esteem in children with visual-motor integration difficulties influences the results of a randomized intervention trial. *Research in developmental disabilities,* 34(1), 56-64 DOI:10.1016/ j.ridd.2012.07.024.

Lorenzini, V. L. (1993). *Uma escala para detectar a disgrafia baseada na escala de Ajuriaguerra* (dissertação de Mestrado) [*A scale for detecting dysgraphia based on the Ajuriaguerra scale* (Master's thesis)]. Universidade Federal de São Carlos, São Carlos, SP.

Martin N. A. *Test of visual perception skills*. 3rd edition. Novato, CA: Academic Therapy Publications; 2006.

McCloskey, M., & Rapp, B. (2017). Developmental dysgraphia: An overview and framework for research. *Cognitive neuropsychology,* 1-18. DOI 10.1080/02643294.2017.1369016.

Milner, D., & Goodale, M. (2006). *The visual brain in action.* US: Oxford University Press.

Okuda, P. M. M., Lourencetti, M. D., Santos, L. C. A. D., Padula, N. A. D. M. R., & Capellini, S. A. (2011). Coordenação motora fina de escolares com dislexia e transtorno do déficit de atenção e hiperatividade [Fine motor coordination of schoolchildren with dyslexia and attention deficit hyperactivity disorder]. *Revista CEFAC,* 13 (5), 876-885.

Pereira, D. M., Araújo, R. D. C. T., & Braccialli, L. M. P. (2011). Relationship Analysis between Visual-Motor Integration Ability and Academic Performance. *Journal of Human Growth and Development*, 21, 808-817. https://doi.org/10.7322/jhgd.20033.

Pontart, V., Bidet-Ildei, C., Lambert, E., Morisset, P., Flouret, L., & Alamargot, D. (2013). Influence of handwriting skills during spelling in primary and lower secondary grades. *Frontiers in psychology*, 4. DOI: 10.3389/fpsyg.2013.00818.

Reid, G., Strnadová, I., & Cumming, T. (2013). Expanding horizons for students with dyslexia in the 21st century: universal design and mobile technology. *Journal of Research in Special Educational Needs*, *13*(3), 175-181. DOI: 10.1111/1471-3802.12013.

Schneck, C. M., Amundson, S. J., Case-Smith, J., & O'Brien, J. C. (2010). Prewriting and handwriting skills. *Occupational therapy for children*, *6*, 555-580.

Tomchek, S. D., & Schneck, C. M. (2006). Evaluation of handwriting. In A. Henderson, & C. Pehoski (Ed.). *Hand Function in the Child* (Second Edition, pp. 291-318). Missouri, EUA: Mosby.

Tseng, M. H., & Chow, S. M. (2000). Perceptual-motor function of school-age children with slow handwriting speed. *American Journal of Occupational Therapy,* 54(1), 83-88. DOI:10.5014/ajot.54.1.83.

Vinter, A., & Chartrel, E. (2010). Effects of different types of learning on handwriting movements in young children. *Learning and instruction*, *20*(6), 476-486.

Zou, K. H., Tuncali, K., & Silverman, S. G. (2003). Correlation and simple linear regression. *Radiology,* 227(3), 617-628. DOI: 10.1148/radiol. 2273011499.

About the Editors

Monique Herrera Cardoso

Affiliation: São Paulo State University "Júlio de Mesquita Filho" – UNESP - Marília- São Paulo – Brazil; Email: moniquehc@gmail.com

Education: Student at Graduate Program in Education, Faculty of Philosophy and Science - FFC – São Paulo State University "Júlio de Mesquita Filho" – UNESP - Marília- São Paulo, Brazil

Research and Professional Experience: PhD Student in the Postgraduate Program in Educationa, Faculty of Philosophy and Science - FFC – São Paulo State University "Júlio de Mesquita Filho" – UNESP – Marília - São Paulo – Brazil. Areas of research: learning disorders, dyslexia, handwriting, ADHD, education, school children.

Professional Appointments: Degree in Speech and Language Pathologist from the Faculty of Philosophy and Science - FFC – São Paulo State University (2009), a Master Degree in Speech and Language Pathologist from the Faculty of Philosophy and Science - FFC – São Paulo State University (2014) Student at Graduate Program in Education, Faculty of

Philosophy and Science - FFC – São Paulo State University "Júlio de Mesquita Filho" – UNESP - Marília- São Paulo – Brazil.

Honors: Special Tribute International - People Expression 2017 - Special category: Best Practices in Education, Brain Connection - II Internacional Congress of Neuroscience and Chilhood and Adolescence Learnig.

Publications Last 3 Years:

Cardoso, M.H.; Capellini, S.A. *Compreendendo os Transtornos específicos de aprendizagem - Compreendendo a disgrafia. 1. ed* [*Understanding Specific Learning Disorders - Understanding Disgrafia. 1. ed.*]. Ribeirão Preto: BookToy, 2017. v. 1. 72p.

Cardoso, M.H.; Capellini, S.A. Speed and Legibility: Brazilian Students Performance in a Thematic Writing Task. In: Byron Leite Dantas Bezerra; Cleber Zanchettin; Alejandro H. Toselli; Giuseppe Pirlo. (Org.). *Handwriting: Recognition, Development and Analysis. 1ed.* Hauppauge, NY: Nova Science Publishers, 2017, v. 1, p. 341-351.

Cardoso, M.H.; Oliveira, A.M. Reading Processes in Students with Attention Deficit Disorder with Hyperactivity. In: Simone Aparecida Capellini; Fábio Henrique Pinheiro; Giseli Donadon Germano. (Org.). *A Handbook of Attention Deficit Hyperactivity Disorder (ADHD) in the Interdisciplinary Perspective. 1 ed.* Sharjah: Bentham Science Publishers, 2016, v. 1, p. 31-40.

Cardoso, M.H.; Capellini, S.A. Identificação e caracterização da disgrafia em escolares com dificuldades e transtornos de aprendizagem. *Distúrbios da Comunicação* [Identification and characterization of dysgraphia in schoolchildren with learning difficulties and disorders. *Communication Disorders*], v. 28, p. 27-37, 2016.

Cardoso, M.H.; Romero, Ana Carla Leite, Capellini, S.A. Alterações de processos fonológicos e índice de gravidade em uma amostra de fala e de escrita de escolares de ensino público e privado. *Psicopedagogia* (São Paulo) [Phonological process changes and severity index in a speech and writing sample of public and private school children. *Psychopedagogy* (São Paulo)], v. 33, p. 283-293, 2016.

Cardoso, M. H.; Uvo, M. F. C.; Capellini, S. A. Perfil de desempenho em habilidades metalinguisticas, leitura e compreensão leitora em escolares do 3o ao 5o ano do ensino público fundamental. In: Olga Valéria Campana dos Anjos Andrade; Paola Matiko Martins Okuda; Simone Aparecida Capellini. (Org.). *Tópicos em Transtornos de Aprendizagem - Parte IV*. 1 ed. [Profile of performance in metalinguistic skills, reading and reading comprehension in students from 3rd to 5th year of fundamental public education. In: Olga Valéria Campana dos Anjos Andrade; Paola Matiko Martins Okuda; Simone Aparecida Capellini. (Org.). *Topics in Learning Disorders - Part IV. 1 ed.*] Marília: Fundepe, 2015, v. IV, p. 19-40.

Sampaio, M.N.; Cardoso, M.H. A produção textual e a interferência da legibilidade e velocidade. In: Olga Valéria Campana dos Anjos Andrade; Paola Matiko Martins Okuda; Simone Aparecida Capellini. (Org.). *Tópicos em Transtornos de Aprendizagem - Parte IV. 1ed.* [The textual production and the interference of readability and speed. In: Olga Valéria Campana dos Anjos Andrade; Paola Matiko Martins Okuda; Simone Aparecida Capellini. (Org.). *Topics in Learning Disorders - Part IV. 1ed.*] Marília: Fundepe, 2015, v. IV, p. 73-88.

Capellini, S.A.; Cardoso, M.H. PTF para intervenção com a função motora fina e escrita. In: Pró-Fono. (Org.). *Planos Terapêuticos Fonoaudiológicos (PTFs). 1ed.* [PTF for intervention with fine and written motor function. In: Pro-Phone. (Org.). *Therapeutic Speech Therapy Plans (PTFs). 1ed.*] Barueri: Pró-Fono, 2015, v. 2, p. 195-202.

Cardoso, M. H.; Henderson, S.; Capellini, S. A. Translation and cultural adaptation of Brazilian Detailed Assessment of Speed of Handwriting: conceptual and semantic equivalence. *Audiology - Communication Research*, v. 19, p. 321-326, 2014.

Simone Aparecida Capellini, PhD

Affiliation: Full-Professor at Department of Speech and Hearing Sciences. São Paulo State University "Júlio de Mesquita Filho" (UNESP), Marília, São Paulo, Brazil. Coordinator at Investigation Learning Disabilities Laboratory (LIDA), Department of Speech and Hearing Sciences, São Paulo State University "Júlio de Mesquita Filho" (UNESP), Marilia, São Paulo, Brazil. Email: sacap@uol.com.br

Education: Speech Language Pathology

Research and Professional Experience:

Dr. Simone Aparecida Capellini has been working the last 13 years as a Professor of the Graduate Program in Education and Graduate Program in Speech Language Pathology at the São Paulo State University "Júlio de Mesquita Filho" (UNESP), Marília, São Paulo, Brazil, where she orients both masters, doctoral and PhD students.

Professional Appointments:

Graduate Program in Education and Graduate Program in Speech Language Pathology at the São Paulo State University "Júlio de Mesquita Filho" (UNESP), Marília, São Paulo, Brazil

Publications Last 3 Years:

Articles published

Uvo, M.F.C.; Germano, Giseli Donadon; Capellini, Simone Aparecida. Desempenho de escolares com transtorno do déficit de atenção com hiperatividade em habilidades metalinguísticas, leitura e compreensão leitora [Performance of schoolchildren with Attention Deficit Hyperactivity Disorder in metalinguistic skills, reading and reading comprehension.]. *Revista CEFAC* (Online), v.19, p.7 - 19, 2017.

Capellini, S.A.; Giaconi, C.; Germano, G.D. Relation between Visual Motor Integration and Handwriting in Students of Elementary School. *Psychology*, v.08, p.258 - 270, 2017.

Germano, G.D.; César, Alexandra Beatriz Portes De Cerquei; Capellini, Simone Aparecida Screening Protocol for Early Identification of Brazilian Children at Risk for Dyslexia. *Frontiers in Psychology*, v.8, p.1 - 13, 2017.

Germano, G.D.; Brito, L. B.; Capellini, S.A. The opinion of parents and teachers of students with learning disorders regarding executive function skills. *Revista CEFAC*, v.19, p.674 - 682, 2017.

Germano, Giseli Donadon; Giaconi, C.; Capellini, S.A. Characterization of Brazilians Students with Dyslexia in Handwriting Proficiency Screening Questionnaire and Handwriting Scale. *Psychology Research*, v.6, p.590 - 597, 2016.

Oliveira, Adriana Marques De; Germano, Giseli Donadon; Capellini, Simone Aparecida. Desempenho de escolares em provas de processo de identificação de letras e do processo léxico [Performance of schoolchildren in the process of identification of letters and the lexical process]. *Revista CEFAC* (Online)., v.18, p.1121 - 1132, 2016.

Germano, Giseli Donadon; Capellini, Simone Aparecida. Identification of Students at Risk for Attention Deficit Disorder with Hyperactivity Using the Response to Intervention Model (RTI). *Psychology* (Irvine)., v.07, p.1824 - 1838, 2016.

Germano, G.D.; Capellini, S.A. Avaliação das habilidades metafonológicas (PROHFON): caracterização e comparação do desempenho em escolares [Evaluation of metaphonological skills (PROHFON): characterization and comparison of performance in schoolchildren]. *Psicologia: Reflexão e Crítica.*, v.28, p.378 - 387, 2015.

Oliveira, Adriana Marques De; Germano, Giseli Donadon; Capellini, Simone Aparecida. Desempenho de escolares com dificuldades de aprendizagem em programa computadorizado de intervenção metafonológica e leitura [Performance of students with learning difficulties in a computerized program of metaphonological intervention and reading]. *Psicologia Argumento* (PUCPR. Impresso)., v.33, p.226 - 241, 2015.

Capellini, Simone Aparecida; César, Alexandra Beatriz Portes De Cerquei; Germano, Giseli Donadon. Early Identification of Reading Problems:

Preliminary Study with Students of 1st Grade. *Procedia: Social and Behavioral Sciences.*, v.174, p.1351 - 1355, 2015.

Fusco, Natália; Germano, Giseli Donadon; Capellini, Simone Aparecida. Efficacy of a perceptual and visual-motor skill intervention program for students with dyslexia. *CoDAS*, v.27, p.128 - 134, 2015.

Oliveira, A.M.; Germano, G.D.; Capellini, S.A. Performance of Brazilian dyslexic students in reading: a comparative study by gender. *Education, Science & Society*, v.6, p.137 - 149, 2015.

Published books

Cerqueira-Cesar, A.B.P.; Germano, G.D.; Capellini, S.A. *Programa de Remediação fonológica para escolares de risco para dislexia (PROF-RD)* [*Phonological Remediation Program for schoolchildren at risk for dyslexia (PROF-RD)*]. Ribeirão Preto: Booktoy, 2018, v.1. p.107.

Capellini, S. A.; Cerqueira-Cesar, A. B. P.; Germano, G.D. *Protocolo de Identificação precoce dos problemas de Leitura – IPPL* [*Early Identification Protocol for Reading Problems - IPPL*]. Ribeirão Preto: Booktoy, 2017, v.1. p.72.

Germano, Giseli Donadon; Capellini, Simone Aparecida. *Protocolo de Avaliação das Habilidades Metafonológicas: Manual de Instrução para aplicação dos Resultados* [*Metaphonological Abilities Assessment Protocol: Instruction Manual for application of Results*]. Ribeirão Preto/SP: Booktoy, 2016, v.1. p.88.

Cardoso, M.H.; Capellini, S.A. *Compreendendo os Transtornos específicos de aprendizagem - Compreendendo a disgrafia. 1. ed.* [*Understanding Specific Learning Disorders - Understanding Disgrafia. 1. ed.*] Ribeirão Preto: Booktoy, 2017. v. 1. 72p.

Book chapters published

Capellini, Simone Aparecida; Santos, B.; Martins, M.A.; Germano, Giseli Donadon. Intervenção fonoaudiológica na dislexia do desenvolvimento In: *Dislexia do Desenvolvimento e Adquiridas.1 ed.* [Speech-Language Intervention in Developmental Dislexia In: *Developmental and Dyslexia Dyslexia.1 ed.*]. São Paulo: Pearson

Clinical Brazil, 2017, v.1, p. 329-341.

Germano, G.D.; Capellini, S.A. Joao, A case study of a Brazilian Adolescent with dyslexia In: *Dyslexia in Adolescence. Global Perspectives.1 ed.* New York: Routledge, 2017, v.1, p. 139-151.

Germano, G.D.; Capellini, S.A. Characterization of Cognitive-Linguistic Profile and Neuroimaging in Attention Deficit Hyperactivity Disorder In: *A Handbook of Attention Deficit Hyperactivity Disorder (ADHD) in the Interdisciplinary Perspective.1 ed.* Sharjah, U.A.E.: Bentham Science Publishers Ltd., 2016, v.1, p. 19-29.

Capellini, Simone Aparecida; Germano, G.D. Dislexia do Desenvolvimento: contribuições das teorias para o diagnóstico e intervenção In: *Neuropsicologia do Desenvolvimento: Infância e adolescência. 1 ed.* [Developmental dyslexia: contributions of theories to diagnosis and intervention In: *Developmental Neuropsychology: Childhood and adolescence. 1 ed.*] Porto Alegre - RS: Artmed, 2016, v.1, p. 125-131.

Germano, G.D.; Liporaci, G.F.S.; Capellini, S.A. Investigation of the Subtypes of Developmental Dyslexia in Brazilian's Children In: *Dyslexia: Perspectives, Challenges and Treatment Options. 1 ed.* USA: Nova Science Publishers Inc., 2016, v.1, p. 117-126.

Cerqueira-Cesar, A.B.P.; Germano, G.D.; Capellini, S.A. O uso do modelo de resposta à intervenção (RTI) para a identificação de escolares de risco para dislexia In: *Tópicos em Transtornos de Aprendizagem - Parte V. 1 ed.* [The use of the intervention response model (RTI) for the identification of schoolchildren at risk for dyslexia In: *Topics in Learning Disorders - Part V. 1 ed.*]. Marília: Fundepe, 2016, v.1, p. 95-108.

Capellini, Simone Aparecida; Giaconi, C.; Germano, G.D. Parents and Teachers Opinion about Learning Skills: Comparison between Brazilian and Italian Dyslexic's Students In: *Dyslexia: Perspectives, Challenges and Treatment Options. 1 ed.* United States of America: Nova Science Publishers Inc., 2016, v.1, p. 91-98.

Capellini, S.A.; Orlandi-Cunha, Vera Lúcia; Germano, Giseli Donadon. Processos de Intervenção com os Transtornos da Leitura e da Escrita:

Diretrizes para a Identificação Precoce e a Remediação Fonoaudiológica In: *Tratado de Linguagem: perspectivas contemporâneas.1 ed.* [Processes of Intervention with Reading and Writing Disorders: Guidelines for Early Identification and Speech-Language Pathology Remediation In: *Language Treatise: Contemporary Perspectives. 1 ed.*] Ribeirão Preto/SP: BookToy, 2016, v.1, p. 233-242.

Uvo, M.F.C.; Germano, G.D.; Capellini, S.A. Relação entre as habilidades metalinguísticas e compreensao de leitura de textos expositivos em escolares com Transtornos do Déficit de Atenção com Hiperatividade In: *Tópicos em Transtornos de Aprendizagem - Parte V. 1 ed.* [Relationship between metalinguistic abilities and reading comprehension of expository texts in schoolchildren with Attention Deficit Hyperactivity Disorder, In: *Topics in Learning Disorders - Part V.1 ed.*] Marília: Fundepe, 2016, v.1, p. 122-135.

Capellini, S.A.; Pinheiro, F.H.; Germano, G.D. *Summary of eBook In: A Handbook of Attention Deficit Hyperactivity Disorder (ADHD) in the Interdisciplinary Perspective. 1 ed.* Sharjah, U.A.E.: Bentham Science Publishers Ltd., 2016, v.1, p. 1-1.

Okuda, P.M.M.; Germano, G.D. Visual Perception of Students with Attention Deficit and Hyperactivity Disorder In: *A Handbook of Attention Deficit Hyperactivity Disorder (ADHD) in the Interdisciplinary Perspective. 1 ed.* Sharjah, U.A.E.: Bentham Science Publishers Ltd., 2016, v.1, p. 57-69.

Germano, G.D.; Capellini, S.A. Avaliação da Leitura e da Escrita na perspectiva fonoaudiológica In: *Abordagem multidisciplinar da aprendizagem. 1 ed.* [Assessment of Reading and Writing in the Speech-Language Pathology Perspective In: *Multidisciplinary approach to learning. 1 ed.*]. Viseu, Portugal: Editora QualConsoante, Ltda, 2015, v.1, p. 519-529.

Capellini, S.A.; Germano, G.D. Characterization and Comparison of performance of studnets with Learning difficulties and good readers from publi and private school in tests of reading and writing of word and pseudowords In: *Private and Public schools - International*

Perspectives, management and educacional efficiency.1 ed. New York: Nova Publishers, 2015, v.1, p. 115-132.

Germano, G.D.; Capellini, S.A. Habilidades metafonológicas em escolares com dislexia do desenvolvimento: implicações educacionais In: *Dislexia: novos temas, novas perspectivas vol III. 1 ed.* [Metaphonological skills in schoolchildren with developmental dyslexia: educational implications In: *Dyslexia: new themes, new perspectives vol III. 1 ed.*] Rio de Janeiro - RJ : Wak Editora, 2015, v.1, p. 45-56.

Germano, G.D.; Okuda, P.M.M. O uso do Modelo de Resposta à Intervenção para identificação precoce do TDAH e TDC In: *Tópicos em Transtornos de Aprendizagem - Parte IV. 1 ed.* [The use of the Intervention Response Model for early identification of ADHD and BDD In: *Topics in Learning Disorders - Part IV. 1 ed.*] Marília - SP: FUNDEPE Editora, 2015, v.1, p. 211-222.

Capellini, S.A.; Silva, E. C.; Germano, Giseli Donadon. O uso do modelo de resposta à Intervenção (RTI) para a identificação do Transtorno do Déficit de Atenção e Hiperatividade In: *Transtorno do Déficit de Atenção/Hiperatividade (TDAH): prática clínica e educacional. 1 ed.* [The use of the Intervention response model (RTI) for the identification of Attention Deficit Hyperactivity Disorder In: *Attention Deficit Hyperactivity Disorder (ADHD): clinical and educational practice. 1 ed.*] Marília - SP: FUNDEPE Editora, 2015, v.1, p. 119-132.

Capellini, Simone Aparecida; GERMANO, Giseli Donadon. Plano Terapêutico Fonoaudiológico (PTF) para remediarão fonologia Associada a Leitura e Escrita In: *Planos Terapêuticos Fonoaudiológicos (PTFs). 1 ed.* [Therapeutic Phonoaudiological Plan (PTF) to remedy phonology Associated with Reading and Writing In: *Speech Therapy Plans (PTFs). 1 ed.*] BaruerI -SP: Pró-Fono, 2015, v.1, p. 223-228.

Cardoso, M.H.; Capellini, S.A. Speed and Legibility: Brazilian Students Performance in a Thematic Writing Task. In: Byron Leite Dantas Bezerra; Cleber Zanchettin; Alejandro H. Toselli; Giuseppe Pirlo.

(Org.). *Handwriting: Recognition, Development and Analysis.* 1ed. Hauppauge, NY: Nova Science Publishers, 2017, v. 1, p. 341-351.

Organized books

Capellini, S.A.; Pinheiro, F. H.; Germano, G.D. *A Handbook of Attention Deficit Hyperactivity Disorder (ADHD) in the Interdisciplinary Perspective.* Sharjah, U.A.E.: Bentham Science Publishers Ltd., 2016, v.1. p.134.

LIST OF CONTRIBUTORS

Juliana Flores Mendonça Alves

Affiliation: Universidade Federal de Minas Gerais, Brazil

Education: Degree in Occupational Therapy UFMG; Graduate degree in Neuroscience from UFMG; 2014-Specialist in Sensory Integration for the WPS California. Master of Rehabilitation Sciences at the UFMG.

Research and Professional Experience:
Collaborator of the Laboratório de Estudos dos Transtornos da Aprendizagem (LETRA) HC/Universidade Federal deMinas Gerais.
Project Extension; LETRAmento e saúde na comunidade-UFMG

Professional Appointments:
2009 – Collaborator of the Laboratório de Estudos dos Transtornos da Aprendizagem (LETRA) HC/Universidade Federal deMinas Gerais;
2010-present – Clinic with approach in child development;
2014-2015 – Substitute professor in occupational therapy-UFMG

Publications Last 3 Years:

Alves, L.M., Siqueira, C.M., Ferreira, M.C.M., Alves, J.F.M., Lodi, D.F., Bicalho, L., Celeste, L. C., (2016). Rapid Naming in Brazilian Students with Dyslexia and Attention Deficit Hyperactivity Disorder. *Frontiers in Psychology*, 7, 1-11.

Alves, J. F. M. (2015). *Adaptação transcultural e análise da validação do Here's How I Write: auto-avaliação da escrita*. Dissertação de mestrado [*Transcultural adaptation and validation analysis of Here's How I Write: self-evaluation of writing*]. Masters dissertation. Programa de Pós Graduação em Ciências da Reabilitação, Universidade de Federal de Minas Gerais, Belo Horizonte.

Siqueira, C.M., Alves, J.F.M., Ferreira, M.C.M., & Alves, L.M. (2015) Baixo desempenho escolar e suas diferentes causas: diagnóstico diferencial. In: Pereira, P.S. (Org.). *Abordagem multidisciplinar de aprendizagem* [*Multidisciplinary approach to learning*]. (pp. 155-178). Lisboa.

Siqueira, C.M., Ferreira, M.C.M., Freitas, E.; Aguiar, J., Alves, J.F.M., Lodi, D. F., Melo, R. M P.A., Franco, L. G.(2015). Transtorno de Déficit de Atenção/Hiperatividade e Transtorno Específico de Aprendizagem - atualizações segundo o Manual de Diagnóstico e Estatístico dos Transtornos Mentais (DSM-5) e suas implicações clínicas. In: Mousinho, R., Alves, L.M., Capellini. S.A. (Org.). *Dislexia: novos temas, novas perspectivas* [*Dyslexia: new themes, new perspectives*]. (pp. 233-250). Rio de Janeiro.

Flores, J.A.M, Siqueira, C. M., Lodi, D.F., Ferreira, M.C.M., ALVES, Alves, L.M., Kummer, A. (2013). Casuística do Laboratório de estudos dos Transtornos de Aprendizagem (LETRA) do Hospital das Clínicas da UFMG. In: Alves, L.M., Mousinho, R., Capellini. S.A. (Org.). *Dislexia - novos temas, novas perspectivas*. [*Dyslexia: new themes, new perspectives*] (257-278) .Rio de Janeiro.

Mirian Aratangy Arnaut, PhD

Affiliation: NEAPEL/University Federal of São Paulo, Brazil

Education: Speech and Language Therapist-University of São Paulo; MSc and PhD Human Communication Disorders – University Federal of São Paulo, Brazil

Research and Professional Experience:
Member of the NEAPEL – Center for Teaching and Research in Reading and Writing – Departament of Speech and Language Pathology - Escola Paulista de Medicina – University Federal of São Paulo. Clinical Speech and Language Therapist.

Professional Appointments:
Speech and Language Graduate at University of São Paulo. MSc and PhD from the Departament of Speech and Language Pathology - University Federal of São Paulo. My object of study is the learning disorders particularly writing mistakes and its relation with the metacognitive mechanisms.

Honors:
Master' s dissertation, Ensurdecimento na fala de crianças disfônicas de 04 a 08 anos *(Voiceless in the speech of dysphonic children aged from 4 to 8 years old)* was awarded at the XIII Brazilian Congress of Speech and Language Pathology, by the Brazilian Society of Speech and Language Pathology, 2004.

Publications Last 3 Years:
Arnaut, Mirian Aratangy; Hackerott, Maria Mercedes Saraiva; Bueno, Gabriela Juliane; Nepomuceno, Pablo Felício; Avila, Clara Regina Brandão. Erros de base fonológica na escrita: codificação de surdas e sonoras, segmentação e juntura vocabular. [Phonological basis mistakes in writing: codification of voiced and voiceless letters,

word segmentation and junction] *Audiology-Communication Research.* 2014.19(3):264-271. ISSN:2317-6431. Doi: 10.1590/S2317-64312014000300010

Roza, Caroline, Soares; Arnaut, Mirian Aratangy; Carvalho, Carolina Alves Ferreira; Kida, Adriana Batista; Avila, Clara Regina Brandão. Correlações entre escrita ortográfica e reconhecimento de palavras em escolares do ensino fundamental [Correlation between orthographic writing and word recognition in primary school children]. *22nd Brazilian Congress of Speech and Language Pathology,* 2014. Anais Joinvile, SC.

Arnaut, Mirian Aratangy; Hackerott, Maria Mercedes Saraiva, Moreira, Hugo Cogo; Avila, Clara Regina Brandão. Analyse Psychometric des items de la dictée - Théorie de Réponses aux Items ITR (Psychometric analysis of dictation items – Items Theory Response) *Writing Research Across Borders*. 2014. Paris, France.

Damasceno, Esmeralda Sandra; Avila, Clara Regina Brandão; Arnaut, Mirian Aratangy. Correlações entre a escrita manual e o desempenho de escolares do Fundamental 1 [Correlation between handwriting and performance of primary school children]. *Distúrbios da Comunicação.* 2015. 27(4):819-830. ISSN:2176-2724.

Clara Regina Brandão de Avila, PhD

Affiliation: Universidade Federal de São Paulo – Escola Paulista de Medicina, Sao Paulo, Brazil

Education: Speech-Language and Hearing Sciences

Research and Professional Experience:

Speech and language pathologist. Associate Professor at Speech–Language and Hearing Sciences Department in Escola Paulista de Medicina – Universidade Federal de São Paulo (EPM-UNIFESP), Brazil. Research group leader whose work focuses on reading and writing process and their connections with auditory processing and oral language development, psycholinguistic and neurocognitive characteristics of learning and language and learning diseases, at preschool and elementary school. Research lab coordinator: Center for Teaching, Assistance and Research in Writing and Reading – NEAPEL/UNIFESP. Assistant and collaborator with other researchers of different departments and clinical areas of UNIFESP as well.

Professional Appointments:

Speech-language and hearing sciences bachelor's degree; Communication Disorders MS (1986); Communication Sciences and Disorders PhD - Universidade Federal de São Paulo (1990). Habilitation. Communication Disorders Sciences - Universidade Federal de São Paulo (2015)

Honors:

Prêmio Melhor Trabalho-Pôster (2017) [Best Work-Poster Award (2017)]: Efeito da simplificação de vocabulário e da legibilidade sobre os diferentes níveis de processamento da compreensão leitora no 1o. e 2o. ciclo do EF, UNESP - Marília - Laboratório de Investigação dos Desvios da Aprendizagem.

Prêmio Menção Honrosa (2016) [Honorable Mention Award (2016)]: Lexical-access in bilingual students using a Rapid Automatized Naming Task, Sociedade Brazileira de Fonoaudiologia

Prêmio Menção Honrosa (2016) [Honorable Mention Award (2016)]: Efeito do bilinguismo sobre a velocidade de evocação de palavras em pré-escolares e escolares, Sociedade Brazileira de Fonoaudiologia

Prêmio Capes de Tese (2013) Medicina II [Capes de Thesis Award (2013) Medicine II], Capes

Prêmio em Fonoaudiologia - Menção Honrosa (2008) [Award in Speech Therapy - Honorable Mention (2008)]: Reconto e respostas a questões abertas na avaliação da compreensão leitora: estudos preliminares, Sociedade Brazileira de Fonoaudiologia

Prêmio Excelência em Fonoaudiologia (2008) [Excellence in Speech Therapy Award (2008)]: Relação entre a função pragmática da linguagem e compreensão de textos, Sociedade Brazileira de Fonoaudiologia

Prêmio Melhor Dissertação de Mestrado (2004) [Best Masters Thesis Award (2004)]: Ensurdecimento na fala de crianças disfônicas de 04 a 08 anos, Sociedade Brazileira de Fonoaudiologia, em 2004

Publications Last 3 Years

Lucio, P.S.; Cogo-Moreira H; Carvalho, C.A.F.; Kida, A.S.B.; Avila, C.R.B. Prova de nomeação rápida de figuras para crianças: evidências de validade e normas intragrupo. *PSICO-USF* (Impresso) [Proof of quick naming of figures for children: evidence of validity and intra-group norms. *PSICO-USF* (Printed)], v. 22, p. 35-47, 2017.

Rossi, S.G.; Hackerott, M.M.S.; Avila, C.R.B. Creation of a list of homonyms in Brazilian Portuguese for linguistic processing tasks. *CoDAS*, v. 29, p. e20160042, 2017.

Bueno, G.J.; Carvalho, C.A.F.; Avila, C.R.B. Capacity for self-monitoring reading comprehension in Elementary School. *CoDAS,* v. 29, p. e20160044-4, 2017.

Isotani, S.M.; Avila, C.R.B.; Puccini, R.F. Mudanças curriculares no Curso de Graduação em Fonoaudiologia da UNIFESP [Curricular changes in the Speech Therapy Course at UNIFESP]. *Distúrb. Comum.* v. 29, p. 237, 2017

Bueno, G.J.; Rossi, S.G.; Appezzato, M.M.; Chang, E.M.; Carvalho, C.A.F.; Kida, A.S.B.; Avila, C.R.B. Interference of phonological disorder on the reading of items with different psycholinguistic characteristics. *Audiol, Commun. Res.* (ACR), v. 22, p. e1692, 2017.

Kida A.S.B., Bueno G.J., Lima V.C.C. Nepomuceno P.F., Rossi S.G., Martin, M.M.M., Avila, C.R.B. Influence of retelling modality on reading comprehension assessment. *Estudos de Psicologia* (Campinas), v. 32, p. 605-615, 2015.

Kida, A.S.B.; Avila, C.R.B.; Capellini, S.A. Reading comprehension assessment through retelling: performance profiles of children with dyslexia and language-based learning disability. *Frontiers in Psychology*, v. 7, p. 787, 2016

Carvalho CAF, Lucio PS, Avila CRB. Psychometric equivalence of the Brazilian version of the Test of Pragmatic Language 2 - TOPL-2. *CoDAS*, v. 27, p. 344-349, 2015.

Cintra, I.P.; Avila, C.R.B.; Komeno, E.M.; Schoen, T.H. Velocidade de leitura e desempenho escolar na última série do ensino fundamental. *Estudos de Psicologia* [Reading speed and school performance in the last grade of elementary school. *Psychology Studies*] (Campinas), v. 32, p. 437-447, 2015.

Avila C.R.B.; Oppenheimer-Fleury, F. Rapid naming, phonological memory and reading fluency in Brazilian bilingual students. *CoDAS*, v. 27, p. 65-72, 2015.

Lucio, P.S.; Kida, A.S.B.; Carvalho, C.A.F.; Cogo-Moreira, H.; Avila, C.R.B.. Construction of a task for assessing reading comprehension in elementary school: pilot study. *Temas Psicol.* v. 23, p. 1035-1050, 2015.

Lima, V.L.C.C.; Grecco, L.A.C.; Marques, V.C.; Fregni, F.; Avila, C.R.B. Transcranial direct current stimulation combined with integrative speech therapy in a child with cerebral palsy: A case report. *Journal of Bodywork and Movement Therapies*, v. 20, p. 252-257, 2015.

Kida, A.S.B.; Avila, C.R.B.; Capellini, S.A. Syntactic markers in the oral retelling of dyslexic students. *CoDAS*, v. 27, p. 557-564, 2015.

Damasceno, E.S.S.; Avila, C.R.B. Correlações entre o traçado da escrita manual e o desempenho ortográfico de escolares do fundamental I. [Correlations between the handwriting tracing and the orthographic performance of elementary school children I] *Distúrbios da Comunicação*, v. 27, p. 819-830, 2015.

Lima, V.L.C.C.; Kida, A.S.B.; Avila, C.R.B. Estimulação cerebral não invasiva nos transtornos do desenvolvimento da linguagem e da fala. In: *Estimulação cerebral não invasiva nos transtornos do desenvolvimento* [*Noninvasive Brain Stimulation in Developmental Disorders*]. Mauro Muszkat; Luanda André Collange Grecco. (Org.). Curitiba: Editora CRV, 2017, v. 1, p. 177-182.

Carvalho, C.A.F.; Avila, C.R.B.; Kida, A.S.B. Compreensão de leitura na Dislexia do Desenvolvimento. In: Salles J.F.; Navas A.L. (Org.). *Dislexia do Desenvolvimento e Adquiridas* [*Dyslexia of Development and Acquired*]. São Paulo: Pearson Clinical Brazil, 2017, v., p. 275-288.

Avila, C.R.B.; Kida, A.S.B.; Carvalho, C.A.F. Avaliação da comunicação mediada pela escrita. In: Dionísia Aparecida Cusin Lamônica; Denise Brandão de Oliveira e Britto. (Org.). *Tratado de linguagem: perspectivas contemporâneas* [*Language deal: contemporary perspectives*]. Ribeirão Preto: BookToy, 2016, v. 1, p. 90-105.

Avila, C.R.B.; Kida, A.S.B; Carvalho, C.A.F. Atuação fonoaudiológica nos transtornos de aprendizagem. In: Bianca dos Santos; Andrea Oliveira Batista; Simone Aparecida Capellini. (Org.). *Tópicos em transtornos de aprendizagem* [*Topics in learning disorders*], parte V. Marília: FUNDEPE Editora, 2016, v. 7, p. 109-121.

Perissinoto, J.; Avila, C.R.B.; Kida, A.S.B.; Armonia, A.C., Chang, E.M. Efeitos da tutela em construção de narrativa oral infantil. In: Lélia Erbolato Melo. (Org.). *Competência pragmática e linguística na leitura de imagens: reflexões interdisciplinares* [*Pragmatic and linguistic competence in reading images: interdisciplinary reflections*]. Curitiba: CRV, 2016, v., p. 41-79.

Avila, C.R.B.; Carvalho, C.A.F.; Kida, A.S.B. Estimulação da consciência fonológica na prática educacional e na clínica fonoaudiológica. In: Renata Mousinho, Luciana Mendonça Alves, Simone Capellini (orgs): *Dislexia: novos temas, novas perspectivas* [*Dyslexia: new themes, new perspectives*]. Rio de Janeiro: WAK Editora, 2015, v. III, p. 63-72.

Carvalho, C.A.F.; Kida, A.S.B.; Avila, C.R.B. A compreensão leitora em uma perspectiva evolutiva. In: Renata Mousinho, Luciana Mendonça Alves, Simone Capellini. (Org.). *Dislexia: novos temas, novas perspectivas* [*Dyslexia: new themes, new perspectives*]. Rio de Janeiro: WAK Editora, 2015, v. III, p. 181-192.

Dr. José Alexandre Bastos

Affiliation: São Jose do Rio Preto Medical School- FAMERP

Education: Professor Doctor

Research and Professional Experience:

- Degree in Medical School, Valença-Rio de Janeiro, Brazil (1973)
- Doctor of Medical Science.
- Head of the Child Neurology Department of the Medical School of São Jose do Rio Preto-SP, Brazil.
- Medical Coordinator of "Projeto Gato de Botas".
- Titular Member of the Child Neurology Brazilian Association and the Brazilian Academy of Neurology.

Professional Appointments: Responsible for the Child neurology service of the Faculty of the Medicine of São José do Rio Preto –SP, Brazil

Publications Last 3 Years:

Bastos, José Alexandre; Cecato, Angela Maria Traldi; Martin, Marielza Regina Ismael; Grecca, Kelly Regina Risso; Pierini, Rafael. The prevalence of developmental dyscalculia in Brazilian public school system. *Arquivos de neuro-Psiquiatria* (on line), v. 74, p. 201-206, 2016.

Bastos, Jose Alexandre. *O Cérebro e a Matemática. Edição do autor* [*The Brain and Mathematics. Author's Edition*].

Rotta, Newra Tellechea; Ohlweiler, Lygia; Riesgo, Rudimar Dos Santos; Bastos, Jose Alexandre, et al. *Transtornos da Aprendizagem: Abordagem Neurobiológica e Multidisciplinar* [*Learning Disorders: Neurobiological and Multidisciplinary Approach*]. Artmed Editora, 2006. p. 195-206, cap 2.

Noemi Del Bianco, PhD

Affiliation: PhD in Human Sciences, Education, University of Macerata, Mcerata, Italy.

Education: Scienze della Formazione, University of Macerata, Macerata, Italy

Professional Appointments:
PhD Students in Human Sciences, Education, University of Macerata, Mcerata, Italy

Publications Last 3 Years:
Giaconi, Catia; Del Bianco, Noemi; Capellini, Simone; Taddei, Arianna. *Curriculum and inclusion: critical issues and redefinition lines*. Education Sciences and Society, v. 8, p. 51-62, 2017.

Ana Amélia Cardoso

Affiliation: Professor at Occupational Therapy Department, Federal University of Minas Gerais, Brazil

Education: Occupational Therapist, Doctor in Rehabilitation Sciences

Research and Professional Experience: Experience in Occupational Therapy, teaching and research, with an emphasis on child development, working on the following topics: learning disorders, developmental coordination disorder, attention deficit and hyperactivity disorder, assessment of child development and performance, sensory integration.

Publications Last 3 Years:

Magalhães, Lívia C.; Cardoso, Ana Amélia; Guimarães, Marina Aguiar Pires; Van Petten, Adriana Maria Valladão Novais. How Can We Make Our Assessment of Motor Ability Relevant Cross-Culturally? *Current Developmental Disorders Reports*, v. 2, p. 157-164, 2015.

Cardoso, Ana Amélia; Magalhães, Livia Castro; Rezende, Marcia Bastos. Motor Skills in Brazilian Children with Developmental Coordination Disorder versus Children with Motor Typical Development. *Occupational Therapy International*, v. 21, p. 176-185, 2014.

Ribeiro, L.C.; Cardoso, A.A. Abordagem Floortime no Tratamento da Criança Autista: Possibilidades de Uso pelo Terapeuta Ocupacional. *Cadernos de Terapia Ocupacional da UFSCar* [Floortime Approach in the Treatment of the Autistic Child: Possibilities of Use by the Occupational Therapist. *UFSCar Occupational Therapy Notebooks*], v. 22, p. 399-408, 2014.

Esmeralda Sandra Santos Damasceno

Affiliation: NEAPEL/University Federal of São Paulo, Brazil

Education: Speech and Language Therapist-Amazon University – UNAMA; Specialization in Language and Speech – University Federal of São Paulo; Master Student – University Federal of São Paulo, Brazil

Research and Professional Experience: Member of NEAPEL – Center for Teaching and Research in Reading and Writing - Department of Speech and Language Pathology – Escola paulista de Medicina- University Federal of São Paulo. Clinical Speech and Language Therapist.

Professional Appointments: Speech and Language Graduate at Amazon University-UNAMA and specialization in Language and Speech at University Federal of São Paulo and Master Student at University Federal of São Paulo. I am interested in studying reading and writing disorders.

Publications Last 3 Years:

Damasceno, Esmeralda Sandra; Avila, Clara Regina Brandão; Arnaut, Mirian Aratangy. Correlações entre a escrita manual e o desempenho de escolares do Fundamental 1 [*Correlation between handwriting and performance of primary school children*]. *Distúrbios da Comunicação.* 2015. 27(4):819-830. ISSN:2176-2724.

Giseli Donadon Germano, PhD

Affiliation: Paulista State University Júlio de Mesquita Filho FFC/UNESP São Paulo, Brazil

Professional Appointments: Associate Professor

Research and Professional Experience:

Associate Professor, Doctor of the Department of Special Education Faculty of Philosophy and Sciences of the Paulista State University Júlio de Mesquita Filho FFC/UNESP. She holds a PhD in Speech and Hearing Sciences from the Faculty of Philosophy and Sciences of the Paulista State University Júlio de Mesquita Filho FFC/UNESP (2005). Master's degree (2008) and PhD (2011) in Education by the Faculty of Philosophy and Sciences of the Paulista State University Júlio de Mesquita Filho FFC/UNESP. Post-Doctorate by the Laboratoire de Psychologie et Neuro-cognition Grenoble/France (CAPES/BEX-3183/13) (2014). PhD in Phonoaudiology (Department of Speech and Hearing Therapy, FFC/UNESP-Marília-SP). Young Research Fellow by the Pro-Rectory of Research FFC/UNESP (PROP- Ed. 005/2014). She has developed activities as Assistant Professor of the Department of Speech and Hearing Therapy, FFC/UNESP-Marília-SP. Speech and Hearing Therapist Collaborating Researcher of the Laboratory of Investigation of Learning Disorders LIDA of the Department of Speech and Hearing Therapy FFC/UNESP-Marília-SP. He has experience in Speech Therapy, with emphasis on Learning, working mainly on the following topics: reading, metaphonological skills assessment, intervention programs, viso-motor perception, dyslexia, dysgraphia, learning disorders and attention deficit hyperactivity disorder.

Publications Last 3 Years:

Uvo, M.F.C.; Germano, Giseli Donadon; Capellini, Simone Aparecida, Desempenho de escolares com transtorno do déficit de atenção com hiperatividade em habilidades metalinguísticas, leitura e compreensão leitora. *Revista CEFAC* (Online), v.19, p.7 - 19, 2017.

Capellini, S.A.; Giaconi, C.; Germano, G.D. Relation between Visual Motor Integration and Handwriting in Students of Elementary School. *Psychology*, v.08, p.258 - 270, 2017.

Germano, G.D.; César, Alexandra Beatriz Portes De Cerquei; Capellini, Simone Aparecida, Screening Protocol for Early Identification of Brazilian Children at Risk for Dyslexia. *Frontiers in Psychology*, v.8, p.1 - 13, 2017.

Germano, G.D.; Brito, L.B.; Capellini, S.A. The opinion of parents and teachers of students with learning disorders regarding executive function skills. *Revista CEFAC*, v.19, p.674 - 682, 2017.

Germano, Giseli Donadon; Giaconi, C.; Capellini, S.A. Characterization of Brazilians Students with Dyslexia in Handwriting Proficiency Screening Questionnaire and Handwriting Scale. *Psychology Research*, v.6, p.590 - 597, 2016.

Oliveira, Adriana Marques De; Germano, Giseli Donadon; Capellini, Simone Aparecida. Desempenho de escolares em provas de processo de identificação de letras e do processo léxico [Performance of schoolchildren in the process of identification of letters and the lexical process]. *Revista CEFAC* (Online), v.18, p.1121 - 1132, 2016.

Germano, Giseli Donadon; Capellini, Simone Aparecida. Identification of Students at Risk for Attention Deficit Disorder with Hyperactivity Using the Response to Intervention Model (RTI). *Psychology* (Irvine), v.07, p.1824 - 1838, 2016.

Germano, G.D.; Capellini, S.A. Avaliação das habilidades metafonológicas (PROHFON): caracterização e comparação do desempenho em escolares [Evaluation of metaphonological skills (PROHFON): characterization and comparison of performance in schoolchildren]. *Psicologia: Reflexão e Crítica*, v.28, p.378 - 387, 2015.

Oliveira, Adriana Marques De; Germano, Giseli Donadon; Capellini, Simone Aparecida. Desempenho de escolares com dificuldades de aprendizagem em programa computadorizado de intervenção metafonológica e leitura [Performance of students with learning difficulties in a computerized program of metaphonological intervention and reading]. *Psicologia Argumento (PUCPR. Impresso)*, v.33, p.226 - 241, 2015.

Capellini, Simone Aparecida; César, Alexandra Beatriz Portes De Cerquei; Germano, Giseli Donadon. Early Identification of Reading Problems: Preliminary Study with Students of 1st Grade. *Procedia: Social and Behavioral Sciences*, v.174, p.1351 - 1355, 2015.

Fusco, Natália; Germano, Giseli Donadon; Capellini, Simone Aparecida. Efficacy of a perceptual and visual-motor skill intervention program for students with dyslexia. *CoDAS*, v.27, p.128 - 134, 2015.

Oliveira, A.M.; Germano, G.D.; Capellini, S.A. Performance of Brazilian dyslexic students in reading: a comparative study by gender. *Education, Science & Society*, v.6, p.137 - 149, 2015.

Published books

Cerqueira-Cesar, A.B.P.; Germano, G.D.; Capellini, S.A. *Programa de Remediação fonológica para escolares de risco para dislexia (PROF-RD) [Phonological Remediation Program for schoolchildren at risk for dyslexia (PROF-RD)]*. Ribeirão Preto: Booktoy, 2018, v.1. p.107.

Capellini, S.A.; Cerqueira-Cesar, A.B.P.; Germano, G.D. *Protocolo de Identificação precoce dos problemas de Leitura – IPPL [Early Identification Protocol for Reading Problems - IPPL]*. Ribeirão Preto: Booktoy, 2017, v.1. p.72.

Germano, Giseli Donadon; Capellini, Simone Aparecida. *Protocolo de Avaliação das Habilidades Metafonológicas: Manual de Instrução para aplicação dos Resultados [Metaphonological Abilities Assessment Protocol: Instruction Manual for application of Results]*.

Ribeirão Preto/SP: Booktoy, 2016, v.1. p.88.

Cardoso, M.H.; Capellini, S.A. *Compreendendo os Transtornos específicos de aprendizagem - Compreendendo a disgrafia. 1. ed.* [*Understanding Specific Learning Disorders - Understanding Disgrafia. 1. ed.*] Ribeirão Preto: BookToy, 2017. v. 1. 72p.

Catia Giaconi

Affiliation: Full Professor of Didactic and Special Pedagogy, Department of Education, Cultural Heritage and Tourism, University of Macerata, Macerata, Italy.

Education: Scienze della Formazione, University of Macerata, Mcerata, Italy

Research and Professional Experience:
Catia Giaconi has been working in the last year as a professor of the Graduate Human Sciences Program, Education, University of Macerata, Mcerata, Italy.

Professional Appointments:
Graduate Human Sciences Program, Education, University of Macerata, Mcerata, Italy.

Publications Last 3 Years:
Articles

Giaconi, Catia; Del Bianco, Noemi; Capellini, Simone; Taddei, Arianna. Curriculum and inclusion: critical issues and redefinition lines. *Education Sciences and Society*, v. 8, p. 51-62, 2017.

Germano, G.D.; Giaconi, C.; Capellini, S.A. Characterization of Brazilians Students with Dyslexia in Handwriting Proficiency Screening Questionnaire and Handwriting Scale. *Psychology Research*, v. 6, p. 590-597, 2016.

Book

Giaconi, C.; Capellini, S.A. *Conoscere per includere: riflessioni e linee operative per professionisti in formazione. 1a. ed.* [*Know to include: reflections and operational guidelines for trainees. 1 bis. ed.*] Milano - Itália: Franco Angelli, 2015. 194p.

Cynthia Y. Hiraga, PhD

Affiliation: São Paulo State University (UNESP), Biosciences Institute, Campus of Rio Claro, Brazil

Education:

Undergraduate Degree in Physical Education, Londrina State University, UEL, Brazil

Master of Science in Human Movement Sciences, São Paulo State University (UNESP), Biosciences Institute, Campus of Rio Claro, Brazil

Doctor of Philosophy in Human Motor Control, University of Tasmania, Australia

Research and Professional Experience:

Research in Human Motor Behavior. Teaching experience at the undergraduate level in neurophysiology, motor development, and motor learning. Teaching experience at the graduate level in research methods.

Professional Appointments:

2007-2010: Assistant Professor at the University of São Paulo, Brazil

2010-present: Assistant Professor at the São Paulo State University (UNESP), Biosciences Institute, Campus of Rio Claro, Brazil

Publications Last 3 Years:

Hiraga, C.Y.; Tonello, M.G.M.; Pellegrini, A.M. Contribution of virtual reality (Nintendo Wii) for exercise training and rehabilitation. In:

Barbieri, F. A. & Vitorio, R. (Org.). *Locomotion and Posture in Older Adults. 1 ed.*: Springer International Publishing, 2017, p. 371-384.

Pasculli, A.G.; Hiraga, C.Y.; Pellegrini, A.M. Tradução transcultural do Minnesota Handwriting Assessment para o contexto Brazileiro. *Cadernos De Terapia Ocupacional Da Ufscar* [Transcultural translation of the Minnesota Handwriting Assessment into the Brazilian context. *Ufscar Occupational Therapy Notebooks*], v. 25, p. 95-104, 2017.

Reis, J.G.; Neiva, C.M.; Pessoa Filho, D.M.; Ciolac, E.G.; Verardi, C.E. L.; Siqueira, L.O.C.; Goncalves, D.F.; Silva, G.R.; Hiraga, C.Y.; Tonello, M. G. M. Virtual Reality Therapy: motor coordination and balance analysis in children and teenagers with Down syndrome. Motricidad. *European Journal of Human Movement*, v. 38, p. 53-67, 2017.

Gama, D.T.; Hiraga, C.Y.; Ferracioli, M.C.; Pellegrini, A.M. *Value of pre-cue information for motor tasks performed by children with developmental coordination disorder (DCD).* Motriz, v. 22, p. 138-143, 2016.

Andrade, V.L.B.; Ferracioli, M.C.; Hiraga, C.Y.; Pasculli, A.G.; Pellegrini, A.M. Efeito da posição do punho no controle de preensão em pinça de adultos jovens. *Cadernos de Terapia Ocupacional da UFSCar* [Effect of wrist position on grip control in young adult tweezers. *UFSCar Occupational Therapy Notebooks*], v. 23, p. 515-523, 2015.

Gabriela Franco dos Santos Liporaci

Affiliation: Investigation Learning Disabilities Laboratory, Departament of Speech and Hearing Sciences, São Paulo State Universty "Júlio de Mesquita Filho" (UNESP), Marília, São Paulo, Brazil.

Education: Speech Language Pathology

Research and Professional Experience:
Research at Investigation Learning Disabilities Laboratory, Departament of Speech and Hearing Sciences, São Paulo State Universty "Júlio de Mesquita Filho" (UNESP), Marília, Brazil. Professional Appointments: Graduate Student in Speech and Hearing Sciences Program

Publications Last 3 Years:
Germano, G.; Liporaci, G.F.S.; Capellini, S.A. Investigation of the subtypes of developmental dyslexia in Brazilian's children. In: Marilyn Frazier. (Org.). *Dyslexia: Perspectives, Challenges and Treatment Options*. In: Marilyn Frazier. (Org.). New York: Nova Science Publishers, Inc., 2016, v. 1, p. 117-126.

Lívia de Castro Magalhães, PhD

Affiliation: Universidade Federal de Minas Gerais, Brazil

Education: Occupational Therapist with a PhD in Education

Research and Professional Experience:
Lívia de Castro Magalhães has been working for the past 15 years as a Professor of the Graduate Program in Rehabilitation Sciences, at the Universidade Federal de Minas Gerais, where she orients both masters and doctoral students.

Professional Appointments: Graduate Program in Rehabilitation Sciences, at the Universidade Federal de Minas Gerais

Publications Last 3 Years:
Dornelas, Lílian De Fátima; Magalhães, Lívia De Castro. Desempenho funcional de escolares que receberam diagnóstico de atraso do desenvolvimento neuropsicomotor até os dois anos [Functional performance of schoolchildren who received a diagnosis of delayed

neuropsychomotor development up to two years]. *Revista Paulista de Pediatria* (Impresso), v.34, p.78 - 85, 2016.

Alves, Caroline De Oliveira; Magalhães, Lívia De Castro; Moreira, Rafaela Silva; Silveira, Isabella Freitas Da; Machado, Márcia Gomes Penido; Viana, Cândida Ferrarez Bouzada. Factors associated with the development of preterm children at four and eight months of corrected gestational age. *Journal of Human Growth and Development*, v.26, p.41 - , 2016.

Dornelas, L.F.; Duarte, N.M.C.; Morales, N.M.O.; Pinto, R.M.C.; Araujo, R.R.H.; Pereira, S.A.; Magalhaes, L.C. Functional Outcome of School Children With History of Global Developmental Delay. *Journal of Child Neurology*, v.31, p.1 - 11, 2016.

Moreira, Tarcísio Santos; Magalhães, Lívia De Castro; Silva, Rafael Duarte; Martin, Robroy L.; Resende, Marcos A. Translation, cross-cultural adaptation and validity of the Brazilian version of the Foot and Ankle Ability Measure questionnaire. *Disability and Rehabilitation*, v.38, p.1 - 12, 2016.

Dornelas, Lílian De Fátima; Duarte, Neuza Maria De Castro; Magalhães, Lívia De Castro. Atraso do desenvolvimento neuropsicomotor: mapa conceitual, definições, usos e limitações do termo [Delay of neuropsychomotor development: conceptual map, definitions, uses and limitations of the term]. *Revista Paulista de Pediatria* (Impresso), v.33, p.88 - 103, 2015.

Garcia, Natalia Barbosa Coronado; Magalhães, Livia De Castro; Santos, Jair Lício Ferreira. Coordenação fina e escrita de crianças de 6 a 9 anos nascidas a termo e pré-termo [Fine and written coordination of 6 to 9 year-old children born to term and preterm]. *Revista de Terapia Ocupacional da Universidade de São Paulo*, v.26, p.166 - 175, 2015.

Dornelas LF; Magalhães, L.C.; Lima, C.G.S.E.; Van Petten, A.M.V.N. Desempenho de crianças nascidas pretermo e em idade escolar na escrita: revisão da literatura [Performance of preterm and school-age children in writing: literature review]. *Cadernos de Terapia Ocupacional da UFSCar.*, v.23, p.177 - 187, 2015.

Oliveira, Suelen Rosa De; Machado, Ana Carolina Cabral De Paula;

Miranda, Débora Marques De; Campos, Flávio Dos Santos; Ribeiro, Cristina Oliveira; Magalhães, Lívia De Castro; Bouzada, Maria Cândida Ferrarez. Espectroscopia de luz próxima ao infravermelho como ferramenta auxiliar no estudo do desenvolvimento infantil [Infrared light spectroscopy as an auxiliary tool in the study of children's development]. *Revista Paulista de Pediatria* (Impresso)., v.33, p.230 - 240, 2015.

De Castro Magalhães, Lívia; Cardoso, Ana Amélia; Guimarães, Marina Aguiar Pires; Van Petten, Adriana Maria Valladão Novais. How Can We Make Our Assessment of Motor AbilityRelevant Cross-Culturally? *Current Developmental Disorders Reports*, v.2, p.101 - , 2015.

Assumpção, Fernanda; Faria-Fortini, Iza; Magalhães, Lívia; Basílio, Marluce; Carvalho, Augusto; Teixeira-Salmela, Luci. Measurement properties of the LIFE-H 3.1-BRAZIL for the assessment of social participation after stroke. *Revista de Neurociências* (EPM. Impresso)., v.23, p.506 - 515, 2015.

Madalena; Assis, Silvana Maria Blascovi; Magalhães, L.C. Modelo lúdIco: Favorecendo o BrIncar da crIança coM deFIcIêncIa FísIca. revista da sobama., v.16, p.15 - 18, 2015.

Cury, Rosane Luiza M; Carvalho, A.M.; Magalhaes, Livia C.; Pinto, P.A. F. Primeira infância e pobreza no Brazil: uma análise integrada a partir de indicadores em saúde, educação e desenvolvimento [Early childhood and poverty in Brazil: an integrated analysis based on health, education and development indicators]. *Revista de Políticas Públicas*., v.19, p.303 - 3014, 2015.

Magalhães, L.C.; Gontijo, A.P.B. Assessing Gross Motor Development of Brazilian Infants. *Pediatric Physical Therapy*, v.26, p.48 - 55, 2014.

Agostini, Olívia Souza; Magalhaes, Livia C.; Campos, A.F. Assessment of motor coordination and dexterity of six years old children: A psychometric analysis. Motriz: *Revista de Educação Física* (Online), v.20, p.167 - 176, 2014.

Moreira, Rafaela S.; Magalhães, Lívia C.; Alves, Claudia R.L. Effect of preterm birth on motor development, behavior, and school performance of school-age children: a systematic review. *Jornal de Pediatria* (Impresso), v.90, p.119 - 134, 2014.

Moreira, Rafaela S.; Magalhães, Lívia C.; Dourado, Jordana S.; Lemos, Stela M.A.; Alves, Claudia R.L. Factors influencing the motor development of prematurely born school-aged children in Brazil. *Research in Developmental Disabilities*, v.35, p.1941 - 1951, 2014.

Magalhães, L.C.; Dunn, L.; Mancini, Marisa C. Internal Structure of the Children Helping Out: Responsibilities, Expectations, and Supports (CHORES) Measure. *The American Journal of Occupational Therapy*., v.68, p.286 - , 2014.

Cardoso, Ana Amélia; Magalhaes, Livia C. Motor Skills in Brazilian Children with Developmental Coordination Disorder versus Children with Motor Typical Development. *Occupational Therapy International*, v.21, p.176 - 185, 2014.

Galvão, B.A.P.; Bueno, K.P.; Rezende, M.B.; Magalhaes, Livia C. Percepção materna do desempenho de crianças com transtorno do desenvolvimento da coordenação [Maternal perception of the performance of children with developmental coordination disorder]. *Psicologia em Estudo* (Impresso)., v.19, p.527 - 538, 2014.

Galvão, B.A.P.; Veloso, M.; Carvalho, L.P.F.; Magalhães, L.C. Perspectiva dos pais sobre as consequências funcionais do Transtorno do Desenvolvimento da Coordenação (TDC): revisão da literatura. *Cadernos de Terapia Ocupacional da UFSCar* [Parents' perspective on the functional consequences of Coordination Developmental Disorder (CDD): literature review. *UFSCar Occupational Therapy Notebooks*], v.22, p.187 - 193, 2014.

Maggi, Eliane F.; Magalhães, Lívia C.; Campos, Alexandre F.; Bouzada, Maria Cândida F. Preterm children have unfavorable motor, cognitive, and functional performance when compared to term children of preschool age. *Jornal de Pediatria* (Impresso), v.90, p.377 - 383, 2014.

Marielza Regina Ismael Martins

Affiliation: São José do Rio Preto Medical School – FAMERP Projeto Gato de Botas – Parceria FAMERP/Secretaria de Educação de São José do Rio Preto/SP

Education: Professor Doctor

Research and Professional Experience: Degree in Occupational Therapy from the Pontifical Catholic University of Campinas (1982), a Master's Degree in Health Sciences from the São José do Rio Preto Medical School (2004) and a PhD in Health Sciences from the São José do Rio Preto Medical School (2007). Occupational Therapist, Department of Neurological Sciences, FAMERP. Areas of research: learning disorders, chronic pain, quality of life.

Professional Appointments: Occupational Therapist of the Department of Neurological Sciences

Publications Last 3 Years:

Forni, J.E.; Rocha, C.E.; Dias, Lilian Chessa; Cunha, Ana Marcia; Araujo Filho, G.M.; Foss, Marcos Daglio; Santos Junior, R.; Martins, Marielza Ismael. Effectiveness of an Interdisciplinary Program on the Limitations and Quality of Life of the Patients with Failed Back Surgery Syndrome. *Coluna/Columna*, v. 16, p. 48, 2017.

Marini, Adriana Maira; Martins, Marielza R. Ismael; Forni, J.E.; Araujo Filho, G.M. Papéis Ocupacionais e Qualidade de Vida em Individuos com dor Crônica. *Ciência Em Movimento- Reabilitação E Saúde* [Occupational Papers and Quality of Life in Individuals with Chronic Pain. *Science in Movement- Rehabilitation and Health*], v. 38, p. 119, 2017.

Martins, M.R.I; Cunha, Ana Marcia Rodrigues da; Dias, Lilian Chessa; Forni, J.E.; Santos Junior, Randolfo dos. Auto percepção da qualidade de vida e identificação da alexitimia em pacientes com síndrome da falha cirúrgica [Self perception of the quality of life and identification of alexithymia in patients with surgical failure syndrome]. *Revista Dor*, v. 18, p. 23, 2017.

Dantas, J.; Martins, Marielza Regina Ismael. Correlação entre dor e qualidade de vida de pacientes hemodialíticos [Correlation between pain and quality of life of hemodialytic patients]. *Revista Dor*, v. 18, p. 124-127, 2017.

Vides, M.; Martins, M.R.I. Avaliacao da dor ossea em pacientes renais cronicos em hemodialise [Evaluation of bone pain in chronic renal patients on hemodialysis]. *Revista Dor*, v. 18, p. 245-248, 2017.

Bastos, José Alexandre; Cecato, Angela Maria Traldi; Martins, Marielza Regina Ismael; Grecca, Kelly Regina Risso; Pierini, Rafael. The prevalence of developmental dyscalculia in Brazilian public school system. *Arquivos de Neuro-Psiquiatria* (Online) JCR, v. 74, p. 201-206, 2016.

Citations ("Web of Science"/Scopus):

Miyahira, Clara Kimie; Martins, Marielza Regina Ismael; Mendonça, Rita De Cassia Helu Ribeiro; Cesarino, Claudia Bernardi. Avaliação Da Dor Torácica, Sono E Qualidade De Vida De Pacientes Com Doença Renal Crônica. *Arquivos de Ciências da Saúde (FAMERP)* [Evaluation of Chest Pain, Sleep, and Quality of Life of Patients With Chronic Kidney Disease. *Archives of Health Sciences (FAMERP)*], v. 23, p. 61, 2016.

Padovani, M.; Martins, M.R.I; Venancio, A.; Forni, J.E. Ansiedade, Depressão E Qualidade De Vida Em Individuos Com Dor Do Membro Fantasma. *Acta Ortopédica Brazileira* (Impresso) [Anxiety, Depression And Quality Of Life In Individuals With Ghost Member Pain. *Brazilian Orthopedic Act* (Printed)], v. 23, p. 107-110, 2015.

Beigin, G.; Martins, Marielza Ismael; Forni, J. E.; Venancio, A. Psychosocial and quality of life impact on patients with failed back surgery syndrome. *Revista Dor*, v. 16, p. 32-36, 2015.

Lace, A.; Marielza Ismael Martins. Conhecimento da atividade motora e fatores clinicos de crianças com Sindrome de Down e a sobrecarga de seus cuidadores. *Arquivos de Ciências da Saúde (FAMERP)* [Knowledge of the motor activity and clinical factors of children with Down syndrome and the overload of their caregivers. *Archives of Health Sciences (FAMERP)*], v. 22, p. 70-74, 2015.

Pereira, Adriana Dos Santos; Carneiro, Caroline Caserta; Pinto, Maria Helena; Martins, Marielza Regina Ismael; Netinho, João Gomes; Cesarino, Claudia Bernardi. Percepções dos estomizados intestinais sobre o estoma após cirurgia [Perceptions of ostomy patients concerning stoma after surgery]. *Ciência, Cuidado e Saúde* (Online), v. 14, p. 1051-1057, 2015.

Martins, Marielza Regina Ismael; Ramos, Leticia Lima; Foss, Marcos Henrique Dáll Aglio; Mansanares De Melo, Silmara Regina; Dias, Lilian Chessa; Santos Junior, Randolfo Dos; Forni, José Eduardo Nogueira; Cunha, Ana Marcia Rodrigues Da; Rocha, Carlos Eduardo D'all Aglio; Laurenti, Mateus Rodrigo. Impacto Funcional Na Qualidade De Vida De Indivíduos Com Síndrome Dolorosa Pós Laminectomia. *Arquivos de Ciências da Saúde (FAMERP)* [Functional Impact on the Quality of Life of Individuals with Painful Post - Laminectomy Syndrome. *Archives of Health Sciences (FAMERP)*], v. 22, p. 41-45, 2015.

Valéria de Cássia Marques

Affiliation: NEAPEL/ University Federal of São Paulo, Brazil

Education: Occupational Therapist - University Federal of São Carlos (UFSCar); Student of the master's program of Human Communication Disorders – University Federal of São Paulo.

Research and Professional Experience: Student of the master's program of Human Communication Disorders, NEAPEL (Center for Teaching and Research in Reading and Writing – Departament of Speech and Language Pathology - Escola Paulista de Medicina – University Federal of São

Paulo. Occupational Therapist - University Federal of São Carlos (UFSCar). Completed master's thesis: "Motor Skills Related to the Acquisition of Manual Writing in Students in the Post-Caligraphc phase", in November 2016.

Professional Appointments: Graduate in Occupational Therapy by University Federal of São Carlos – UFSCar, Student of the master's program of Human Communication Disorders, NEAPEL (Center for Teaching and Research in Reading and Writing – Department of Speech and Language Pathology – Escola Paulista de Medicina – University Federal of São Paulo. My object of study is Typical Motor Development an Atypical, and an Analysis of Movements and Functions employed in Writing.

Publications Last 3 Years:

Grecco, L.C.; Duarte, N.A.C.; Oliveira, C.S.; Muszkat, M.; Zanon, N.; Marques, V.C. Transcranial direct current stimulation combined with motor therapy in children with cerebral palsy classified on level IV oh the GMFCS: A case series. *Gait & Posture*, v. 49/S2, p. 34, 2016.

Carvalho Lima, Vania L.C.; Collange Grecco, Luanda A.; Marques, Valéria C.; Fregni, Felipe; Brandão de Ávila, Clara R. Transcranial direct current stimulation combined with integrative speech therapy in a child with cerebral palsy: A case report. *Journal of Bodywork and Movement Therapies*, v. 20, p. 252-257, 2016.

Adriane Guzman Pasculli Milani

Affiliation: São Paulo State University (UNESP), Biosciences Institute, Campus of Rio Claro, Brazil

Education:

Undergraduate Degree in Occupational Therapy, São Paulo State University (Unesp), School of Philosophy and Sciences, Marília, Brazil

Specialization in Hand Therapy and Rehabilitation of Upper Limbs, Federal University of São Carlos, São Carlos, Brazil

Master of Science in Human Development and Technologies, São Paulo State University (UNESP), Biosciences Institute, Campus of Rio Claro, Brazil

Research and Professional Experience: Research in Human Motor Behavior.

Professional Appointments:

2011 - Current Occupational Therapist of the Municipal Health Foundation of Rio Claro.

Publications Last 3 Years:

Pasculli, A.G.; Hiraga, C.Y.; Pellegrini, A.M. Tradução transcultural do Minnesota Handwriting Assessment para o contexto Brazileiro. *Cadernos de Terapia Ocupacional da Ufscar* [Transcultural translation of the Minnesota Handwriting Assessment for the Brazilian context. *Ufscar Occupational Therapy notebooks*], v. 25, p. 95-104, 2017.

Andrade, V.L.B.; Ferracioli, M.C.; Hiraga, C.Y.; Pasculli, A.G.; Pellegrini, A.M. Efeito da posição do punho no controle de preensão em pinça de adultos jovens. *Cadernos de Terapia Ocupacional da UFSCar* [Effect of wrist position on grip control in young adult tweezers. *UFSCar Occupational Therapy Notebooks*], v. 23, p. 515-523, 2015.

Ana Maria Pellegrini, PhD

Affiliation: São Paulo State University (UNESP), Biosciences Institute, Campus of Rio Claro, Brazil

Education:

Undergraduate Degree in Physical Education and Pedagogy, University of São Paulo, USP, Brazil

Master of Science in Kinesiology, University of Illinois, C-U, USA
Doctor of Philosophy in Kinesiology, University of Illinois, C-U, USA

Research and Professional Experience:

Research in Human Motor Behavior. Teaching experience at the undergraduate level in motor learning and motor control. Teaching experience at the graduate level in motor development

Professional Appointments:

1968-1986 Assistant Professor at the University of São Paulo

1986-2014 Full Professor (retired) at the São Paulo State University (UNESP), Biosciences Institute, Campus of Rio Claro, Brazil

Honors:

1989 Award Sports Literature granted by the Ministry of Education and Culture

2006 Premio "Jefferson Canfield" granted by the Brazilian Society of Motor Behavior

Publications Last 3 Years:

Hiraga, C. Y.; Tonello, M. G. M.; Pellegrini, A. M. Contribution of virtual reality (Nintendo Wii) for exercise training and rehabilitation. In: Barbieri, F. A. & Vitorio, R. (Org.). *Locomotion and Posture in Older Adults. 1ed.*: Springer International Publishing, 2017, p. 371-384.

Pasculli, A. G.; Hiraga, C. Y.; Pellegrini, A. M. Tradução transcultural do Minnesota Handwriting Assessment para o contexto Brazileiro. *Cadernos de Terapia Ocupacional da Ufscar* [Transcultural translation of the Minnesota Handwriting Assessment for the Brazilian context. *Ufscar Occupational Therapy notebooks*], v. 25, p. 95-104, 2017.

Gama, D. T.; Hiraga, C. Y.; Ferracioli, M. C.; Pellegrini, A. M. Value of pre-cue information for motor tasks performed by children with developmental coordination disorder (DCD). *Motriz*, v. 22, p. 138-143, 2016.

Andrade, V. L. B.; Ferracioli, M. C.; Hiraga, C. Y.; Pasculli, A. G.; Pellegrini, A. M. Efeito da posição do punho no controle de preensão em pinça de adultos jovens. *Cadernos de Terapia Ocupacional da UFSCar* [Effect of wrist position on grip control in young adult tweezers. *UFSCar Occupational Therapy Notebooks*], v. 23, p. 515-523, 2015.

Natália Lemes dos Santos

Affiliation: Faculty of Philosophy and Sciences, São Paulo State University- UNESP - Marília, SP, Brazil.

Education: Undergraduate in Speech Language Pathology Course from Faculty of Philosophy and Sciences, São Paulo State University- UNESP - Marília, SP, Brazil. Will be concluded in 2019.

Flávia Santana Serrão

Affiliation: Investigation Learning Disabilities Laboratory, Departament of Speech and Hearing Sciences, São Paulo State Universty "Júlio de MesquitaFilho" (UNESP), Marília, São Paulo, Brazil.

Education: Speech Language Pathology

Research and Professional Experience: Research at Investigation Learning Disabilities Laboratory, Departamentof Speech and Hearing Sciences, São Paulo State Universty "Júlio de Mesquita Filho" (UNESP), Marília, Brazil.

Professional Appointments: Undergraduate at Speech Language Pathology Course at Faculty of Philosophy and Sciences, State University of São Paulo "Júlio de Mesquita Filho" - FFC - UNESP - Marília (SP), Brazil.

Adriana Maria Valladão Novais Van Petten, PhD

Affiliation: Professor of Occupational Therapy Department, Universidade Federal de Minas Gerais, Brazil

Education: Occupational Therapist, Master and PhD in Mechanical Engineering

Research and Professional Experience: Research and Experience in Occupational Therapy, acting on the following subjects: orthosis, performance evaluation, assistive technology, development of alternative materials for orthosis, desenvolvimento humano/activity and participation, inclusion and accessibility in higher education.

Publications Last 3 Years:

Medeiros, J.S.S.; Dornelas, L.F.; Lima, C.G.S.E.; Van Petten, Amvn; Magalhaes, L.C. Desempenho de crianças nascidas pretermo e em idade escolar na escrita: revisão da literatura. *Cadernos de Terapia Ocupacional da UFSCar* [Performance of preterm and school-age children in writing: literature review. *UFSCar Occupational Therapy Notebooks*], v. 23, p. 177-187, 2015.

Ferreira, F.M.R.; Bortolus, M.V.; Nolasco, A.L.; Melo, E. R.; Viotti, M.B.; Lopes, R.M.; Van Petten, A.M.V.N. Suporte de Leitura: desenvolvimento de um protótipo para auxílio a pessoas com baixa visão - testes preliminares. *Revista de Terapia Ocupacional da Universidade de São Paulo* [Reading Support: development of a prototype to assist people with low vision - preliminary tests. *Occupational Therapy Journal of the University of São Paulo*], v. 26, p. 288, 2015.

Magalhaes, L.C.; Cardoso, A.A.; Guimaraes, M.A.P.; Van Petten, A.M.V.N. How Can We Make Our Assessment of Motor Ability Relevant Cross-Culturally? *Current Developmental Disorders Reports*, p. 1-8, 2015.

Sousa, L.; Rezende, A.; Van Petten, A.M.V.N. *Revista de Terapia Ocupacional da Universidade de São Paulo* [*Occupational Therapy Journal of the University of São Paulo*], v. 26, p. 250-257, 2015.

Van Petten, A.M.V.N; Ávila, A.F.; Girundi, C. *Cadernos de Terapia Ocupacional da UFSCar*, v. 22, p. 79-87, 2014.

Carvalho, M.G.R.; Ávila, A.F.; Van Petten, A.M.V.N. *Revista Iberoamericana de Polímeros*, v. 12, p. 13-22, 2011.

Van Petten, Amvn; Ávila, A. F. Effect of the use of wrist orthosis on forearm muscle activation. *Revista Brazileira de Ortopedia* (Impresso), v. 45, p. 73-80, 2010.

Index

A

B

C

D

I

J

L

M

N

O

P

R

S

V